100 Questions & An About Uterine Fibr

Lloyd B. Greig, MD

Obstetrician/Gynecologist
Department of Obstetrics and Gynecology
The Cedars Sinai Medical Group
Beverly Hills, CA

JONES AND BARTLETT PUBLISHERS
Sudbury, Massachusetts

World Headquarters
Jones and Bartlett Publishers
40 Tall Pine Drive
Sudbury, MA 01776
978-443-5000
info@jbpub.com
www.jbpub.com

Jones and Bartlett Publishers
Canada
6339 Ormindale Way
Mississauga, Ontario L5V 1J2
Canada

Jones and Bartlett Publishers
International
Barb House, Barb Mews
London W6 7PA
United Kingdom

Jones and Bartlett's books and products are available through most bookstores and online book-sellers. To contact Jones and Bartlett Publishers directly, call 800-832-0034, fax 978-443-8000, or visit our website, www.jbpub.com.

Substantial discounts on bulk quantities of Jones and Bartlett's publications are available to corporations, professional associations, and other qualified organizations. For details and specific discount information, contact the special sales department at Jones and Bartlett via the above contact information or send an email to specialsales@jbpub.com.

The authors, editor, and publisher have made every effort to provide accurate information. However, they are not responsible for errors, omissions, or for any outcomes related to the use of the contents of this book and take no responsibility for the use of the products and procedures described. Treatments and side effects described in this book may not be applicable to all people; likewise, some people may require a dose or experience a side effect that is not described herein. Drugs and medical devices are discussed that may have limited availability controlled by the Food and Drug Administration (FDA) for use only in a research study or clinical trial. Research, clinical practice, and government regulations often change the accepted standard in this field. When consideration is being given to use of any drug in the clinical setting, the healthcare provider or reader is responsible for determining FDA status of the drug, reading the package insert, and reviewing prescribing information for the most up-to-date recommendations on dose, precautions, and contraindications, and determining the appropriate usage for the product. This is especially important in the case of drugs that are new or seldom used.

Production Credits
Executive Publisher: Christopher Davis
Editorial Assistant: Sara Cameron
Production Director: Amy Rose
Associate Production Editor: Laura Almozara
Senior Marketing Manager: Barb Bartoszek
V.P., Manufacturing and Inventory Control: Therese Connell
Composition: Glyph International
Cover Design: Colleen Lamy
Cover Images: Top photo: © Brett Rabideau/ShutterStock, Inc.; Bottom left photo:
  © Photos.com; Bottom right photo: © Photodisc
Printing and Binding: Malloy, Inc.
Cover Printing: Malloy, Inc.

Library of Congress Cataloging-in-Publication Data
Greig, Lloyd B.
  100 questions and answers about uterine fibroids / Lloyd B. Greig.
    p. cm.
  Includes bibliographical references and index.
  ISBN-13: 978-0-7637-4639-1
  ISBN-10: 0-7637-4639-8
  1. Uterine fibroids—Popular works. 2. Uterine fibroids—Miscellanea. I. Title.
II. Title: One hundred questions and answers about uterine fibroids.
  RC280.U8G745 2010
  616.99'366—dc22
                                    2009019552

6048

Printed in the United States of America
14 13 12 11 10   10 9 8 7 6 5 4 3 2 1

To my wife, Sally, and our daughters, Tanya and Gabrielle.

Contents

Acknowledgments

I would like to express my gratitude to Ms. Aida Diaz-Winch and Danielle Blum, CNM, RNP, MSN, for their assistance in creating this book, and to Dr. Karyn Morse and Dr. Ronald Leuchter for their objective reviews of the manuscript.

When I began writing this book, my goal was simple—I wanted to provide information on uterine fibroids that was concise, straightforward, accurate, and informative. The language has been kept simple and interesting.

The glossary has a number of medical terms that are not included in the book. These were added to assist the patient in her search for useful information.

I hope I have achieved my goal.

PART ONE

The Basics

What are fibroids?

Are there different types of fibroids?

How are fibroids diagnosed?

More . . .

1. What are fibroids?

Uterine fibroids are benign tumors that can develop:

- Within the uterine cavity
- Within the muscular wall of the **uterus**
- On the surface of the uterus

They are the single most common reason for **hysterectomies** in the United States. It is estimated that between 200,000 to 500,000 hysterectomies are performed each year because of fibroid tumors. Fibroids are the most common noncancerous tumor in women of reproductive age. They are the source of a broad spectrum of pelvic problems, which range from chronic pain to excessive and unpredictable uterine bleeding.

2. Are fibroids known by other names?

They are known interchangeably as fibroids, fibromyomas, leiomyomas, or just plain old myomas. They can vary from the size of a pea to larger than a basketball (**Figure 1**). Decades ago, when women were less likely to seek medical attention for pelvic disorders, doctors frequently saw fibroids that were the size of full-term pregnancies.

You may find it surprising when your **gynecologist** first describes the size of your fibroid in the terms of a growing fetus. Your doctor may tell you that your fibroid is the size of a 12-, 14-, or 17-week pregnancy. The largest fibroid ever removed is reported to have weighed an astounding 140 pounds!

3. What symptoms are usually caused by fibroids?

Because fibroids can grow anywhere in the uterus and in a wide variety of sizes, they are associated with a

Uterine fibroids
Benign tumors that can cause severe abnormal bleeding and extreme pain. Also known as fibromyoma, leiomyoma, and myoma. They may trigger heavy menstrual bleeding, disabling cramps, unpredictable bleeding between periods, and may underlie serious anemia and exhaustion.

Fibroids are the most common noncancerous tumor in women of reproductive age.

Uterus
Also called the womb. This is a pear-shaped hollow organ about three inches long and two inches wide at its top. It has a role in the monthly menstrual cycle, provides an environment for the growth and nourishment of a developing fetus, and produces mild contractile waves as part of the female sexual response.

Hysterectomy
The surgical removal of the uterus.

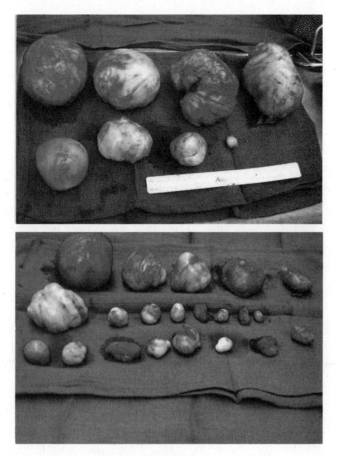

Figure 1   Fibroids ranging in size and shape.

Gynecologist

A medical doctor who has completed a residency specializing in disorders of the female reproductive tract and issues involving endocrinology and reproductive physiology.

Pelvic pressure

A sensation of fullness in the abdomen that can be caused by fibroids.

Anemia

A disorder in which there is a low red blood cell count so the red blood cells carry less oxygen. Anemia can result in fatigue and exhaustion and if left untreated, may be life-threatening.

variety of uterine problems. Their growth may cause abnormal bleeding, **pelvic pressure**, increase in abdominal girth, and pain. Associated symptoms include **anemia** (due to excessive or prolonged bleeding), frequent urination because of pressure on the bladder, problems with bowel movements, as well as pain during sexual intercourse.

The most frequent symptoms that cause women to seek medical attention are abnormal, heavy uterine bleeding and increased pelvic pressure. Symptoms in decreasing order of frequency are:

1. **Abnormal uterine bleeding**
2. Pelvic pressure due to the increasing size of the fibroid(s)
3. Pain

An estimated 30% of women with fibroids experience abnormal uterine bleeding that usually does not begin as extreme blood loss. The build-up to very heavy periods may occur over several months and may lead to severe anemia. In some instances, large clots may occur along with the bleeding.

Patients also report a feeling of "fullness" or pelvic pressure. Fibroid pressure on the bladder may lead to **urinary incontinence**. This pressure may be so severe that some women are forced to wear padding to prevent embarrassment. These benign tumors can also cause hemorrhoids, due presumably to fibroid-induced pressure on the rectal area. Fecal incontinence may affect some women, while constipation is a problem for others.

Pain, which is usually caused by the softening or degeneration of the fibroids, is an infrequently occurring symptom.

If you are experiencing any of these symptoms, you should contact your gynecologist and undergo a full workup for your symptoms.

Scientists at the National Institutes of Health estimate that anywhere from 50% to 80% of women will develop one or more fibroid tumors by the time they reach their

Abnormal uterine bleeding

A disorder caused by any one of several underlying reproductive system conditions; characterized by excessive bleeding and/or blood clots that may lead to anemia.

Urinary incontinence

An inability to prevent the excretion of urine.

35th birthday. Curiously, even after all of the troublesome symptoms are taken into account, only 25% of patients diagnosed with fibroids experience problems serious enough to seek medical treatment. Just as fibroids may prove to be painful nuisances in some women, they are painless and quiescent in others, and their presence is known only after they are discovered during a routine pelvic examination. Indeed, a majority of women with fibroids never report adverse symptoms.

A majority of women with fibroids never report adverse symptoms.

Pam's comment:

In the spring of 1993 at the age of 35, I began to experience extreme pain in my lower abdomen and was having heavier than normal menstrual cycles. As the pain intensified and the bleeding became abnormal, I began to seek answers.

Deborah's comment:

In addition to the incessant bleeding, the symptom that was most aggravating to me was the frequent urination that occurred while I was ovulating. There were several days within each month, prior to my menses, in which I would awaken to go to the bathroom at least 6–10 times during the night.

Cancer
Any malignant development caused by abnormal and uncontrolled growth of cells. Some cancers grow rapidly and invade surrounding tissues and organs; others are more indolent and grow slowly.

4. Why are fibroids called tumors? Can they become cancerous?

Although fibroids are called tumors, these growths are usually composed of benign cells. When they reach sufficient sizes, fibroids can put pressure on other organs or distort the shape of the uterus. Studies have shown that it is rare for a fibroid to become **cancerous**. Those that do, however, develop into the type of malignancy known as a **sarcoma**. U.S. health statistics show that less than 1% of fibroids become cancerous.

Studies have shown that it is rare for a fibroid to become cancerous.

Sarcoma
A highly malignant type of tumor; connective tissue neoplasm.

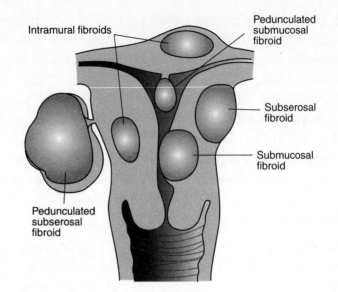

Figure 2   Fibroids in the uterus.

Serosa

Thin outer layer that covers the uterus.

Subserosal fibroids

Fibroids located beneath the outer covering or outer layer (serosa) of the uterus.

Intramural fibroids

A type of fibroid that grows between the smooth muscular walls of the uterus. It may cause symptoms similar to those of submucosal and subserosal fibroids.

Submucosal fibroids

A type of fibroid tumor that develops directly beneath the surface of the endometrium. The large number of blood vessels on its surface can bleed and trigger pain. These fibroids tend to prevent the uterine muscle's ability to properly contract because they distort the shape and function of the organ. They can grow to a size that obstructs the fallopian tubes and also may distort the uterine lining as they grow, causing menstrual irregularities. They may even become pedunculated and project into the cervix or vagina.

5. Are there different types of fibroids?

Fibroids are generally named based on their location in specific areas of the uterus (**Figure 2**). The symptoms that they cause are usually associated with their location.

The different types are as follows:

- **Subserosal fibroids**: The thin layer covering the outside of the uterus is called the **serosa**. Fibroids occurring just below this layer are called **subserosal fibroids**. They may appear as small bumps or large growths on the surface of the uterus.
- **Intramural fibroids**: These are located within the muscular walls of the uterus. They may extend outward to include the subserosal area. It is not unusual to find fibroids that are both subserosal and intramural.
- **Submucosal fibroids**: The lining of the cavity of the uterus is called the mucosa or **endometrium**. Fibroids that are located entirely within the uterine cavity are

called submucosal fibroids. Sometimes an intramural fibroid may extend into the uterine cavity and will therefore have a submucosal component. The submucosal fibroid is the major cause of abnormal uterine bleeding associated with fibroids.

- **Pedunculated fibroids**: A fibroid may extend from a stalk or pedicle and is then called a pedunculated fibroid. They may occur either on the outside or serosal surface of the uterus or in the cavity or mucosal layer of the uterus.

- **Transmural fibroids**: These extend throughout the thickness of the muscular wall of the uterus and may impinge on both the cavity and the external uterine surface.

6. Why do women develop fibroids?

Very little is known about the cause of uterine fibroid tumors, although scientists have suggested several provocative theories. Unfortunately, none fully explains why fibroids develop, let alone why some remain harmless and others become such renegades and sources of both physical and emotional pain. Recent studies have suggested that hormones, the environment, and genetics may be underlying causes, but no one knows for sure. Clinicians have long recognized that fibroid growth is intimately linked with the secretion of **estrogen**. When women reach menopause and ovarian hormone production declines, fibroids tend to shrink dramatically, and in many women, they even disappear. But some scientists contend that the estrogen link may be more associated with the growth of fibroids as opposed to what makes them develop in the first place. While some experts have said the tumors tend to grow in women who produce higher than normal levels of estrogen, laboratory tests have shown that

Endometrium

The inner lining of the uterus.

Pedunculated fibroids

A type of fibroid that grows on a stalk usually on the outside of the uterus.

Transmural fibroids

Fibroids are located within the muscular wall of the uterus. Some of the larger fibroids may extend from the innermost layer (submucosa) of the uterus to the outermost layer (serosa). These would be described as transmural fibroids, which have a submucosal and a subserosal component.

Estrogen

A hormone formed by the ovaries, the placenta during pregnancy, and, to a lesser extent, fat cells with the aid of an enzyme called aromatase. Estrogen stimulates secondary sex characteristics, such as the growth of breasts, and exerts systemic effects (i.e., growth and maturation of long bones and control of the menstrual cycle).

some women whose estrogen secretion is clearly within normal ranges also develop the growths. Scientists are vigorously searching for clues about the origin, growth, and ultimate shrinkage of fibroid tumors. If enough clues are found, medical scientists believe they will be able to piece together a sketchy outline of the natural history of fibroid tumors. Already, at least one prominent clue has surfaced. It involves recent discoveries about certain proteins found in fibroid cells. These discoveries may ultimately help scientists unveil further information about how fibroids seed themselves in the uterus and then grow under the influence of estrogen. Researchers in the reproductive endocrinology division of the National Institutes of Health have found that fibroids have very low levels of a key structural protein that helps hold normal tissue in place. The protein is called **dermatopontin** and it is a major chemical component your body makes to prevent cells from straying into aberrant patterns of growth. In a healthy uterus, adequate supplies of dermatopontin help maintain the integrity of the organ by keeping uterine cells where they are supposed to be.

Fibroids and similar benign growths (such as keloids, which are a type of thick tissue that forms after an incision or wound) tend to have low levels of dermatopontin. A lack of sufficient supplies of the protein may explain why a small portion of the uterus inexplicably develops a fibrous nodule that, over time, can grow until it reaches the size of a golf ball or even a cantaloupe and becomes what is known as a fibroid tumor. If you were to view fibroid tissue under the microscope, you would notice that its very low levels of dermatopontin cause the tumors to have very disorganized and unstructured strands of collagen. Aside from that feature and the very fact that fibroids tend to have low

Dermatopontin

A protein made by the body to prevent cells from staying into aberrant patterns of growth. Researchers have associated low levels of the protein with the development of fibroid tumors.

levels of dermatopontin, scientists have yet to discover other roles that the protein may have in the uterus, Studies of this important chemical component in uterine cells, however, are continuing.

Meanwhile, scientists at the National Institute of Environmental Health Sciences have been researching whether chemical compounds in the environment, mostly pesticides, are capable of mimicking estrogen. If so, scientists are asking whether these chemicals are linked to the development of fibroids and other reproductive system disorders, such as **endometriosis**. Estrogen-like compounds are common in the environment and some scientists have theorized that these chemicals compete with your body's natural estrogen for sites on your cells known as estrogen receptors. It is theorized, but not yet proven, that once a fake estrogen molecule latches onto an estrogen receptor, it can not only block natural estrogen, but it may also unlock the cell and serve as the fuel that drives its growth. The result, the theory holds, may be abnormal growth, such as what your doctor detects in the case of fibroids and other female reproductive system disorders.

Endometriosis

A reproductive system disorder in which tissue from the inner lining of the uterus grows in places it should not be. Endometrial tissue can implant itself anywhere in the pelvic area (including the ovaries, bladder, and large intestine), leading to scar tissue and pain during sexual intercourse and bowel movements. Some patients report a constant dull pain in the abdomen, and an escalation in the degree of pain during menstruation.

Doctors have also long known that women with first-degree relatives diagnosed with the growths are more likely to have fibroids themselves. Problematic fibroids are often seen among relatives, and this observation has had an influence on hysterectomies that have occurred over multiple generations in families. Many American women may feel the necessity to have hysterectomies based on their mothers' or other relatives' experiences. Scientists at the National Institutes of Health (NIH) estimate that, while vast numbers of women develop uterine fibroid tumors, about 75% of patients who are diagnosed with them never experience symptoms.

7. *What is the incidence of fibroids in the United States?*

The prevalence of fibroids varies between 20% and 80% of women in the childbearing range. African American females have the highest incidence of fibroids. These tumors are found to a lesser extent in Caucasian, Asian, and Latina women.

8. *How are fibroids diagnosed?*

As with any medical condition, your physician will begin by taking a detailed medical history. You will be asked a number of specific questions about your:

Menstruation

A discharge of blood, secretions, and tissue fragments from the uterus at regular intervals, usually after ovulation.

- General health
- Previous pregnancies (if any)
- **Menstrual** history
- Experience with abnormal bleeding, pain, or other reproductive system issues
- Diet
- Previous illnesses
- Exercise and health-related conditions that run in your family

Bimanual examination

A type of investigation used for diagnosis, in which the physician places two lubricated gloved fingers into the vagina and pushes upward while also pressing down with the other hand on the outside of the lower abdomen. This action allows the gynecologist to feel any growths in the uterus or on the ovaries.

As part of your diagnostic workup, the doctor will perform a thorough pelvic examination, which will include both a bimanual and a rectovaginal examination. Neither of these procedures should be strange to you because they are the exams your doctor normally conducts during your annual gynecological visit.

9. *What is a bimanual examination?*

Vagina

The passageway from outside of the body to the interior of the reproductive system.

In the **bimanual examination**, your physician places one or two lubricated gloved fingers into the **vagina**, while pressing on the lower abdomen with the other hand.

This action allows the doctor to evaluate the size, position, and shape of the uterus and both ovaries.

10. What is a rectovaginal exam, and is it necessary?

In the **rectovaginal exam**, your doctor places one lubricated gloved finger in the vagina and another in the rectum. Pressure is usually applied on the lower abdomen at the same time. This procedure allows the doctor to further evaluate the ovaries, the back of the uterus, the space behind the uterus, and the rectum.

11. What other tests are done to diagnose fibroids?

A **pelvic ultrasound**, performed either abdominally or transvaginally, is the gold standard for confirming the diagnosis of uterine fibroids. The **ultrasound** is used to determine the location, size, and number of fibroids. The ultrasound, performed repeatedly over a number of months, is also useful in monitoring the rate of growth of uterine fibroids.

Magnetic resonance imaging (MRI) is another useful tool in the diagnosis of fibroids. Computerized tomography (CT) scan has also been used in the diagnosis of fibroids.

12. Why do fibroids cause abnormal uterine bleeding?

More than any other fibroid-related complaint, abnormal uterine bleeding is the reason most women visit their doctors. Abnormal uterine bleeding is also the underlying reason many women with fibroid tumors choose to have hysterectomies. Excessive bleeding may be linked to one of the least common types of fibroids,

Rectovaginal examination

A type of investigation used for diagnosis, in which the physician simultaneously places one lubricated gloved finger in the vagina and another in the rectum. This is an important test for pelvic abnormalities.

Pelvic ultrasound

A machine that utilizes ultrasonic waves to take pictures of the uterus, fallopian tubes, and ovaries, and is used as a diagnostic tool by the doctor. The diagnostic pictures may be taken through the abdomen or through the vagina.

Ultrasound

A type of imaging machine that use high frequency sound waves for medical diagnoses.

called a submucous or submucosal fibroid. Regardless of the term used, the type of growth is the same. This kind of fibroid tumor develops directly beneath the surface of the endometrium. Even though submucosal fibroids may not be as common as their cousin fibroids that grow in other parts of the uterus, they are the cause of the most trouble.

Submucosal fibroids not only are associated with abnormal uterine bleeding, they also have been linked to miscarriages and complica- tions of pregnancy.

Submucosal fibroids not only are associated with abnormal uterine bleeding, they have also been linked to miscarriages and complications of pregnancy. If you are anemic, have experienced several months of pro- longed menstrual bleeding, and are known to have fibroids, a submucosal fibroid may be the type of fibroid (or fibroids) you have. Of course, your physician will extensively evaluate you before arriving at this diagnosis because there are other causes of uterine bleeding.

When your physician examines you for the possible presence of a submucosal fibroid, she or he also will want to rule out any other possible cause of abnormal bleeding, such as ovarian or colorectal cancer. In addi- tion to a manual pelvic examination, your doctor will want a **biopsy** of your endometrial tissue. A biopsy removes tissue so that the cells can be viewed under a microscope. Imaging tests, such as a sonogram, also help your doctor reach a diagnosis.

Biopsy

A surgical procedure in which a tiny sample of tissue is removed so that the cells can be viewed under a microscope and analyzed.

Unlike fibroids that develop in other positions on or inside the uterus, submucosal fibroids tend to have a substantial number of blood vessels on their surfaces that can bleed. They also tend to prevent the uterine muscle from properly contracting because they distort the shape and function of the organ. Another note- worthy feature of submucosal fibroids is their ability to grow large enough to obstruct the **fallopian tubes**, thus preventing passage of an egg in its journey to the uterus. But the story does not end there. These fibroids distort the uterine lining as they grow, causing menstrual irregularities. They may even become pedunculated and project into the **cervix** or even the vagina. As this growth moves about, because it is on a stalk and can twist and turn, it becomes a source of pain as well as abnormal bleeding. It is common for doctors to diagnose and remove submucosal fibroids that are the size of tennis balls.

Submucosal fibroids present many dilemmas for women and their doctors. They can be removed individually in a surgery called a **myomectomy,** or the fibroid and the uterus can be removed together in a hysterectomy. Hysterectomies have been recommended when women have multiple submucosal fibroids or excessive uterine bleeding.

The Basics

Fallopian tubes

Also known as the oviducts. Located at the top part of the uterus (the fundus), the fallopian tubes are the conduits through which eggs cells (ova) are transported to the uterus. At their uppermost ends, the tubes have fingerlike projections that sweep eggs from the ovaries. Each tube measures about four inches in length and possesses contractile capability, a motion that allows them to propel an egg into the uterus.

Cervix

The neck at the lower end of the uterus. It connects the uterus to the vagina. The cervix dilates during labor to allow the birth of a baby.

Myomectomy

A type of surgery used to remove an individual fibroid.

PART TWO

Fibroids and Pregnancy

Do fibroids affect my ability to become pregnant
and to have children?

Do fibroids affect the mother during pregnancy?

How may fibroids affect the baby during pregnancy?

More . . .

13. Do fibroids affect my ability to become pregnant and to have children?

The chief basis for fibroid tumors affecting fertility is location, location, location. Submucosal fibroids (located in the endometrial cavity of the uterus) have been shown to cause the greatest problems with conceiving and also have the strongest association with reduced rates in maintaining a pregnancy. Studies suggest that submucosal fibroids create problems with the implantation of the pregnancy in the uterine cavity, as well as with the location and development of the placenta.

One study showed a 70% decrease in the pregnancy rate of women with submucosal fibroids. Most fertility specialists have been recommending the surgical removal of submucosal fibroids before attempting assisted reproductive techniques such as in vitro fertilization (IVF).

Intramural and subserosal fibroids may adversely affect a woman's ability to become pregnant if they are located near enough to where the fallopian tubes attach to the uterus that they cause an occlusion or blockage of the tubes.

14. Which fibroids are the least likely to cause problems with fertility?

Pedunculated fibroids, attached to the exterior of the uterus, have not been shown to have any adverse effects on fertility. This class of particular fibroids are connected to the surface of the uterus by a narrow stalk or stem. The adverse effect on fertility is in-creased when the fibroids are located in the muscular wall of the uterus or within the cavity or inner chamber of the uterus.

Subserosal fibroids, which are generally located just beneath the outer covering of the uterus, have very little adverse affect on fertility, unless they are located close enough to the fallopian tube to cause compression and blockage.

15. What is the relationship between fibroids and miscarriages?

Several studies have shown a direct relationship between the presence of uterine fibroids and a significant increase in the rate of miscarriages. Submucosal fibroids, and to a lesser extent intramural fibroids, have repeatedly been implicated. One study in particular, which reviewed published reports from 1957 to 1970, showed a significant lowering of miscarriage rates from 41% to 19% in women who had surgical removal of the symptomatic fibroids prior to attempting conception. Essentially, myomectomy (surgical removal of fibroids) significantly decreases the miscarriage rate.

16. Do fibroids affect the mother during pregnancy?

Pain is the most frequently reported symptom or complaint associated with uterine fibroids during pregnancy. At times the fibroid is not diagnosed until after the patient presents with severe pain.

The pain may be intense enough to lead to the patient being hospitalized. However, studies suggest that the pain usually responds to ibuprofen. It should be emphasized that the class of drugs to which ibuprofen belongs—i.e., **nonsteroidal anti-inflammatory drugs (NSAIDs)**—are usually not recommended during the third trimester due to significant potential risks to the baby.

Pain is the most frequently reported symptom or complaint associated with uterine fibroids during pregnancy.

Nonsteroidal anti-inflammatory drugs (NSAIDs)

A group of medications (aspirin, ibuprofen, and naproxen) that reduce inflammation and simultaneously affect the natural hormone-like fatty acids known as prostaglandins, which are a major source of pain and inflammation.

The pain is thought to be due in part to swelling (edema) and infarction (decrease in the blood supply) to the affected fibroid.

The size of the growing uterus may at times be exaggerated by the presence of large fibroids. The increased weight and size may cause difficulty in sleeping, walking, and breathing.

17. How may fibroids affect the baby during pregnancy?

The following list describes how fibroids relate to a few of the more common pregnancy complications:

- Preterm delivery has been shown by several studies to be the leading cause of newborn problems (neonatal morbidity) in pregnancies complicated by uterine fibroids. Preterm delivery may be caused, in part, by an increased incidence of pain in pregnant patients with fibroids.
- Intrauterine growth restriction (IUGR) has not been shown to be a significant problem in pregnancies with fibroids.
- Malposition of the baby is a risk for some pregnant women with fibroids. Specifically, multiple or large fibroids seem to be related to an increase in breeches and/or transverse positions of the baby in the uterus. It is thought that this risk may be due to the fibroids impinging on the space needed for the normal growth and movement of the fetus.
- Placental abruption (premature separation of the placenta) rarely occurs in pregnancies with fibroids, although some studies suggest that patients with fibroids may be at a higher risk for placental abruption.

18. Do fibroids affect the method of delivery of the baby?

Several studies have shown that the presence of fibroids in pregnancy tends to lead to an increased rate of cesarean section deliveries. Cesarean section rates have been reported in the range of 50% in pregnancies with fibroids. The primary reason for the surgical delivery (cesarean section) appears to be malpresentation (e.g., breech) of the baby.

Other studies have demonstrated that vaginal deliveries occur in most pregnancies with fibroids (even large fibroids).

19. What effects may fibroids have on the mother after delivery of the baby?

Postpartum hemorrhage (very heavy bleeding after delivery) is the most common complication with fibroids. This condition is caused, presumably, by the decreased ability of the uterus to contract because of the presence of fibroids. Postpartum hemorrhage may, infrequently, lead to an increase in the rate of emergency hysterectomies.

20. Do fibroids have any effect on the rate of retained placenta?

Retained placenta (afterbirth) is a rare complication of pregnancy. Fibroids have not been shown to have any significant effect on the rate of retained placenta.

21. Is the rate or risk of postpartum infection affected by fibroids?

Fibroids do not appear to have any effect on the rate or the risk of postpartum infection.

PART THREE

Initial Treatment

Should fibroids be treated?

Should I have specific goals before beginning treatment?

Do I need a second opinion before beginning treatment?

More . . .

The frequency and severity of symptoms caused by fibroids may vary quite significantly in each affected woman. The ultimate decision regarding the need for treatment and the options available for treatment is very important.

22. Should fibroids be treated?

Fibroids are essentially benign or noncancerous growths in the uterus. If they are not causing any problems or if the symptoms (e.g., bleeding, pain) are mild, then treatment might not be necessary—or it may be postponed. Your doctor may recommend more frequent examinations to keep track of the fibroids that are affecting you.

23. When does treatment for fibroids become necessary?

Because fibroids can grow anywhere in the uterus and in a wide range of sizes, they are associated with a variety of uterine problems. The growths are most notable for triggering heavy menstrual bleeding, disabling cramps, and unpredictable bleeding between periods, and they may underlie serious anemia and exhaustion resulting from blood loss. An estimated 30% of women with fibroids experience abnormal uterine bleeding that usually does not begin as extreme blood loss. For most, the build-up to very heavy periods occurs gradually over many months until the flow is persistent. In some cases, the blood loss leads to severe anemia, becoming life-threatening. Some women with fibroids report they never seem to stop menstruating, that one period seems to flow into the next. In some instances, large clots may occur along with the bleeding. As fibroids continue to grow, so do the problems. As previously noted, additional concerns include miscarriages and infertility.

Guidelines from the American College of Obstetricians and Gynecologists strongly emphasize that treatment of uterine fibroids be avoided unless the growths are producing symptoms that interfere with the quality of life. While it is prudent to get a proper diagnosis of your fibroid(s), you should not expect to undergo treatment unless the condition is causing abnormal uterine bleeding, severe pain, miscarriages, interference with conception, or incontinence (fecal or urinary). Medical scientists have developed several alternative treatments to hysterectomy for women with problematic fibroid tumors, which will be discussed in greater detail elsewhere in this section. You may find it interesting to note that despite a growing amount of study devoted to fibroid tumors by medical scientists around the world, the growths still pose numerous research questions and a host of medical mysteries.

While it is prudent to get a proper diagnosis of your fibroid(s), you should not expect to undergo treatment unless the condition is causing abnormal uterine bleeding, severe pain, miscarriages, interference with conception, or incontinence.

24. Should I have specific goals before beginning treatment?

It is very important that during discussions with your doctor and before you begin treatment you have a clear understanding of what to expect from the planned method of treatment. It is imperative that both you and your doctor agree that the expectations and goals are realistic. To achieve this, you should be fully informed of all the logical options that are available for treatment.

25. Should I do my own research to learn more about fibroids?

In addition to the information provided by your doctor, you should explore all available sources for additional information. The Internet is generally a useful source of information, but one must be aware that not all information found on the web is reliable. With this information, you will be able to more fully discuss the problem with your doctor and to ask more direct questions.

26. Do I need a second opinion before beginning treatment?

You should always get a second opinion before selecting any method of treatment. Consulting another doctor may increase your knowledge on the subject or may suggest options that were not previously discussed.

27. Should I tell my doctor that I will be seeking a second opinion?

Your doctor should have no objection to your seeking a second opinion. In most cases, your doctor will strongly suggest that you receive second opinions before starting treatment.

28. How do I select a doctor for a second opinion?

There are several sources available:

- You may ask your primary care physician to suggest a doctor.
- You may ask friends or family for suggestions.
- Your insurance company may be able to supply the necessary information.
- Your doctor (gynecologist) may give you the names of some doctors from whom you may get a second opinion.

PART FOUR

Nonsurgical Treatment

Has hormone therapy been used in the treatment of fibroids?

How effective is the Lupron treatment for fibroids?

Are any other medications available for treating fibroids?

More . . .

29. Has hormone therapy been used in the treatment of fibroids?

There is a class of drugs, called **gonadotropin-releasing hormone (GnRH) agonists**, that has been used as a nonsurgical treatment option for fibroids. The most commonly used medications in this class are buserelin, leuprolide, and nafarelin, with leuprolide (Lupron) being the best known. These drugs act by effectively lowering the levels of the female hormones estrogen and **progesterone**. These drugs are therefore effective in decreasing the size of the fibroid and reducing the amount of bleeding associated with fibroids.

30. Are there any side effects with hormonal therapy?

The most common side effects are menopause-related symptoms. These include hot flashes, flushes, mood swings, and irritability. Another worrisome adverse effect is the loss of bone mineral density. These side effects may be reduced by adding estrogen and progesterone to the treatment program. In addition, a significant and substantial regrowth of the fibroids occurs immediately after the hormonal therapy is stopped.

31. How long is the course of treatment with Lupron?

The general effective course may last from 1 to 6 months. The medication is available in 1-month or 3-month injectable doses. The length of therapy may depend on several factors, including:

• The size of your fibroid(s)
• The severity of your symptoms
• The affect on vaginal bleeding

Gonadotrophin-releasing hormone agonists (GnRHa)
A group of medications that prevents the body from making estrogen and progesterone. These medications can be prescribed to help to reduce the size of fibroid tumors by creating a state of pseudo-menopause.

Progesterone
A sex hormone that prepares the uterus for pregnancy.

A significant and substantial regrowth of the fibroids occurs immediately after the hormonal therapy is stopped.

- The timing of additional (surgical) therapy
- The severity of the side effects

32. How effective is the Lupron treatment for fibroids?

Clinical studies have shown the following results:

- Approximately 80% of patients had significantly reduced vaginal bleeding.
- Approximately 60% showed a decrease of 25% in the size of the uterus.
- Approximately 50% of patients had a 25% reduction in the size of the fibroids.
- Pelvic and abdominal pressure was decreased.
- Pelvic and abdominal pain was decreased or relieved.

33. Am I a candidate for the use of Lupron and similar drugs?

There is a specific guideline to determine if you are a candidate to this type of therapy. You should NOT take this medication if you are:

1. Pregnant
2. Breast-feeding
3. Allergic to any of the ingredients of the Lupron class of drugs
4. Having any abnormal uterine bleeding that has not been definitively diagnosed

34. Are the Lupron class of drugs expensive?

These hormonal medications are usually covered, partially or entirely, by most insurance companies. Most health maintenance organizations (HMOs) provide coverage for this class of medications and also provide information of a general nature on this method of treatment.

Mifepristone

A synthetic steroid hormone that blocks the action of progesterone. It is used in a few small studies of women with fibroids and is capable of slowing or sometimes stopping fibroid growth.

If pain, especially during the menstrual period, is the only symptom, over-the-counter pain medication or prescription drugs have been found to be helpful.

Birth control pills

Hormone-based drugs used primarily to prevent conception. Also used as treatments for fibroids and other reproductive system disorders.

35. Are any other medications available for treating fibroids?

A class of antiestrogen and antiprogesterone medications, such as RU-486 (**mifepristone**), has been used on an experimental basis with promising results. It is presently felt that additional studies are needed before these drugs can be recommended.

If pain, especially during the menstrual period, is the only symptom, over-the-counter pain medication or prescription drugs have been found to be helpful.

With heavy bleeding as the chief symptom, oral contraceptives (e.g., **birth control pills**), the birth control injection (Depo-Provera), the patch, or the progesterone-containing intrauterine device (IUD) may be useful.

36. How do these birth control pills and devices help in controlling uterine bleeding?

They control heavy bleeding by reducing (thinning) the thickness of the inner lining of the uterus. They can be helpful even if you do not desire birth control. The following groups of women should NOT use these hormonal treatments:

1. Women with a history of blood clots in their legs
2. Women with a history of blood clots in their lungs
3. Women with a history of breast cancer
4. Women over 35 years of age who are smokers

37. Is the hormone-containing IUD used in the treatment of abnormal bleeding?

The IUD called Mirena contains the progesterone hormone levonorgestrel. It has been shown to substantially reduce menstrual bleeding and has been effective in controlling the abnormal bleeding caused by fibroids in some patients.

38. Are there any new developments for the treatment of fibroids?

One of the newest methods of treatment is called magnetic resonance guided focused ultrasound (MRGFU). This procedure uses high-intensity, focused ultrasound waves to destroy the fibroid.

The benefits of this procedure are:

1. It is noninvasive.
2. No surgery is performed.
3. There is no bleeding.
4. There is no pain.
5. If it is performed as an outpatient procedure, the patient may go home after it is done.

The procedure requires the patient to lie face-down with her abdomen on the ultrasound scanner. The ultrasound scanner is then placed underneath the abdomen and directly below the fibroid. The ultrasound beam is then directed through the wall of the abdomen directly into the fibroid. High-intensity ultrasound energy directed at the fibroid heats the tissue and destroys the fibroid.

39. Are there any potential complications with magnetic resonance guided focused ultrasound (MRGFU)?

Potential side effects include:

- Fever
- Skin burns—The area of skin above the fibroids (on the abdomen) must be adequately shaved before the procedure to prevent skin burns.

- Injury to the bladder or intestines—MRI is used to ensure that these organs are not in the field of treatment.
- Nerve palsy—Pretreatment MRI location is used to prevent damage to nerves.

40. Is MRGFU approved by the Food and Drug Administration (FDA)?

MRGFU is FDA approved for treating uterine fibroids. Although FDA approval was granted in October 2004, this procedure is still regarded by some insurers as new and experimental.

41. Are there holistic or herbal therapeutic options for uterine fibroids?

Review of the alternative medical literature reveals several suggested therapies for fibroids. Some of the suggested guidelines and treatments include:

- Diet—No meat, dairy, or gluten
- Herbs to help shrink fibroids—Ceanothus (red root), fraxinus (white ash), and vitex (chasteberry)
- Nutraceuticals—Vitamin A, B, C, and E
- Minerals—Selenium, calcium, magnesium, zinc, and iron
- Exercise
- Herbs for symptoms
  - Bleeding—Red raspberry and black cohosh
  - Pain, Back cramps—Blue and black cohosh
- Pelvic energy flow—Yoga, acupuncture, tai chi, and qigong
- Meditation

It is suggested that the holistic approach used in conjunction with conventional therapy has shown promising results.

PART FIVE

Surgical Treatment

Does the use of additional medical treatment result in better surgical outcomes?

If I have fibroids and wish to become pregnant, will the surgical removal of the fibroids increase my chances of conceiving?

If the fibroids are not causing any problems, is watchful waiting a better option than surgery?

More . . .

42. Does the use of additional medical treatment result in better surgical outcomes?

Medical treatment may be given before the surgery and during the surgery. Gonadotropin-releasing hormone (GnRH) agonists (such as Lupron) are frequently used for preoperative treatment of fibroids. These drugs have been used for both myomectomy and hysterectomy and have proven very effective in stopping uterine bleeding and causing uterine shrinkage.

The American College of Obstetricians and Gynecologists (ACOG) Practice Bulletin states that GnRH agonists (like Lupron) are the only drugs available that result in clinically significant uterine shrinkage and amenorrhea. On the positive side, these medications do the following:

• Decrease the size of the fibroids
• Decrease the bleeding
• Shorten the hospital stay
• Shorten operating time
• Decrease postoperative pain

On the other hand, these drugs are expensive and have significant side effects.

Also of note, intraoperative medication, such as vasopressin, when injected into the uterine muscle, significantly decreases blood loss during myomectomy.

43. If I have fibroids and wish to become pregnant, will the surgical removal of the fibroids increase my chances of conceiving?

Studies have shown that when fibroids distort the uterine cavity, there is significant adverse effect on fertility due to the decreased implantation rate. Myomectomies (surgical removal of the fibroids) may increase the chances of becoming pregnant by as much as 60%.

44. If the fibroids are not causing any problems, is watchful waiting a better option than surgery?

Generally speaking, observation may be the more prudent course if the fibroids are not causing any problems. On the other hand, if the fibroids show a rapid increase in size, even without any symptoms, it is customarily felt that this may be a warning sign that they may be malignant (cancerous). Surgery is then the indicated course of treatment.

In women who are planning pregnancy, the presence of asymptomatic fibroids, which may be affecting their ability to conceive, usually indicates surgical intervention.

Carolyn's comment:

I had known about my fibroid since discovering it in my first ultrasound when I was pregnant with my son. It was quite small and didn't cause me any discomfort, so no one worried about it. While it was monitored from time to time over the last 8 years, it wasn't until recently that it really became a problem. Suddenly it was large enough to distort my whole abdominal area. I could feel the edges as far as my belly button! I was experiencing a lot of pressure, had more frequent urges to urinate, and just did not feel like myself. The medical opinion was that the fibroid needed to be removed.

45. In women with symptomatic fibroids who are hoping to get pregnant, is surgery a better option than observation?

The more practical and prudent course would be to plan surgery (myomectomy) as close to the desired pregnancy as possible, considering the recurrence rate of fibroids (approximately 25%) after myomectomy. There is also the potential risk of postoperative **adhesion** after myomectomy and the possible adverse effect it may have on fertility. Adhesions tend to develop at the site of previous surgery (i.e., the area from which fibroids were surgically removed). Scarring develops in these areas, which can cause the adjacent organs (intestines, fallopian tubes, and **ovaries**) to become attached. This may lead to blockage of the tubes, swelling or inflammation of the tubes, and subsequently decreased fertility.

46. I have heard my doctors use two terms, laparoscopy and laparotomy. What is the difference?

A **laparoscope** is an important device in the diagnosis and treatment of uterine fibroids and other reproductive system disorders. The instrument allows your surgeon to view your pelvic organs through a keyhole incision in the abdomen. The laparoscope also can aid surgery.

A laparotomy, on the other hand, is an open surgery involving an incision that is made through the abdominal wall either to conduct surgery or to inspect the condition of the pelvic organs. In instances when fibroids are especially large or have grown in a complicated fashion, your doctor may recommend a laparotomy to help preserve the integrity of the uterus, if you are considering a myomectomy (see Part 7).

Adhesion

Fibrous bands of tissue that abnormally cling to nearby structures. They may cause major structures (e.g., ovary, outer walls of the uterus and bladder) to become stuck together. The condition produces extraordinary pain.

Ovary

Twin oval-shaped glands about the size of an almond. They are located on either side of the uterus and contain thousands of ova, also known as germ cells. One egg is released per month, starting at puberty and continuing in a clocklike pattern throughout most of the reproductive years.

Laparoscope

A very small, thin surgical instrument that allows inspection of the abdominal organs through a tiny camera attached to the device.

Pam's comment:

My doctor performed a laparotomy at Cedars-Sinai in order to remove the fibroid tumor, leaving my uterus and fallopian tubes intact. The following year, I developed fibroid tumors again and required another surgery. In order to eliminate the bleeding, I tried birth control pills on my doctor's recommendation. The pills were not an option for me due to my constant nausea. The next fibroid that developed required a laparoscopic procedure in order to alleviate the problem.

PART SIX

Uterine Artery Embolization

What is uterine artery embolization (UAE)?

What are some of the complications of UAE?

What type of evaluation should a patient have to determine if she is a candidate for UAE?

More . . .

47. What is uterine artery embolization (UAE)?

Uterine artery embolization
A surgical technique that blocks the blood supply to problematic fibroids.

Uterine artery embolization, also called uterine fibroid embolization (UFE), was initially used in the 1970s and was subsequently approved in 1995 as a safe and acceptable method for treating uterine fibroids. The procedure is explained in greater detail in Question 60.

By significantly reducing the fibroids' blood supply, the intended result is shrinkage of the growths. A key benefit of the procedure, outside of its potential to alleviate abnormal bleeding, is that it leaves the uterus intact. If you have heard about UAE and think it may be an option worth considering, you will first want to fully discuss the procedure with your healthcare provider to find out if you would be a good candidate. There are numerous reasons some women are not considered for the procedure, as discussed in the following questions.

48. Which women are potential candidates for UAE?

Women who present with symptoms of bleeding, pelvic or abdominal pain, pelvic pressure, increased abdominal girth, or urinary frequency are generally potential candidates for UAE. The size and type of fibroids are also important considerations in selecting patients for this procedure.

49. Which patients are NOT suitable candidates for UAE?

The size of the fibroid is a very important factor. UAE is not very effective in treating fibroids that are 20-weeks' size or larger. The smaller fibroids respond much better. Also, the type of fibroid you have is a significant consideration for this treatment option (as described in Question 50).

Some patients may be allergic to the dyes or contrast media used in UAE. These groups of patients are not candidates for UAE.

50. What are some of the complications of UAE?

When the fibroid is attached to the uterus by a small stalk (pedunculated), the success rate is adversely affected. Moreover, pedunculated fibroids located in the cavity of the uterus (submucosal fibroids), do not respond well to UAE. These fibroids may become detached after embolization, and difficulty is usually experienced in passing or expelling the fibroids.

Patients who have been treated with Lupron (leupro-lide) may also have problems with UAE. Lupron may cause spasms of the blood vessels, which would lead to difficulty in passing a catheter through the blood vessel.

51. What type of evaluation should a patient have to determine if she is a candidate for UAE?

The evaluation should initially include a thorough medical history and physical examination. This examination should include a Pap smear, unless one has been done recently. A complete blood count may also be clinically indicated.

An endometrial biopsy (biopsy of the inner lining of the uterus) should be performed on patients with a history of abnormal uterus bleeding. The endometrial biopsy helps to determine that an underlying malignancy (cancer) is not being overlooked.

An MRI, which is the best method currently available for diagnosing fibroids, is usually recommended in most hospitals, before UAE is performed. The MRI is done even if a pelvic ultrasound was previously performed, as the MRI gives more detailed information.

52. What information should my doctor provide when recommending UAE as an option?

Your doctor should briefly explain how the procedure is performed. He or she should also discuss the success and failure rates, as well as potential complications. Your doctor should also discuss the potential effects of UAE on your ability to become pregnant, as well as the effects on later pregnancies.

53. What else should I know about UAE?

You should be informed of the following:

UAE is a safe option in the treatment of fibroids.

Interventional radiologist
A medical doctor who has completed a residency in radiology and post-residency training in interventional radiology.

- UAE is a safe option in the treatment of fibroids.
- This procedure is performed by an **interventional radiologist**, to whom you will be referred. This doctor will discuss all aspects of the procedure with you in advance.
- UAE is not generally regarded as a surgical procedure and is generally safer than the major surgical treatment options for fibroids (i.e., myomectomy or hysterectomy).
- You should be able to return to work in 7 to 10 days.

54. What will I experience during the UAE procedure?

The procedure of UAE usually takes about 30 minutes from start to finish. Anesthesia, usually very light, is used, making the experience pain free. The level of anesthesia is tailored to the needs of the patient.

The doctor performing the UAE procedure will explain, in detail, the technique involved. He or she will also explain the potential risks involved and will answer all your questions before and after the procedure.

Pam's comment:

My stay in the hospital after my UFE was overnight (23 hours), and the recovery was only a few days at home. Most women return to work after 1 week instead of the 8 weeks required recovering from surgery.

55. What should my realistic expectations be for this procedure?

Within 3 months, most patients experience significant improvement in their symptoms. About 90% of patients show a dramatic improvement in bleeding problems.

56. What should I expect in the first few days after the procedure?

You may experience some mild to moderate abdominal pain immediately after the procedure. Some patients have much more severe abdominal pain and may be hospitalized for 24 to 48 hours for pain management.

A small number of patients may require hospitalization for the first 24 hours after the procedure. This is done, if needed, to control pain. Generally the abdominal cramps respond very well to pain pills.

Pam's comment:

The pain was excruciating following the procedure; however, I was given pain medication to relieve the symptoms.

Also, I was very nauseous, but that passed quickly with medication the following day. The UFE was a much easier procedure for me to manage, and I would recommend it to any woman who is battling fibroid tumors but does not want a partial or full hysterectomy.

57. I have heard of post-embolization syndrome. What is it?

Post-embolization syndrome occurs within the first 24 hours after an embolization has been performed. The patients experience severe pelvic pain, nausea, cramping, and a mild fever. The symptoms are thought to be secondary to the onset of necrosis on tissue destruction in the fibroids. The treatment usually involves:

- Hospitalization for approximately 24 hours,
- Pain management, and
- Treatment for nausea.

This is usually followed by prescribing Motrin or a similar drug for 10 to 14 days and the symptoms usually clear up during that time.

58. When can I expect to return to work following UAE?

Most women are able to return to work in about 7 to 10 days. You will be advised to postpone any excessive physical activity for about 2 weeks.

59. What other adverse reactions might I expect?

The most common adverse reaction is an allergic reaction or rash. Most of these reactions are caused by medications and respond to treatment. Urinary tract infection, injury to the artery, uterine infection, and blood clots have been reported but are very rare. Bleeding and persistent vaginal discharge may also occur.

Adverse reactions, such as infections, may lead to hysterectomy in less than 1% of cases.

A small number of patients may experience expulsion or passing of a fibroid through the vagina following UAE.

60. How is UAE performed?

The procedure is initiated through the patient's femoral artery, which is accessed in the thigh. The doctor cleans the appropriate area on the selected thigh and then places sterile drapes over the area. The patient has an intravenous fluid (IV) line inserted in one arm before the procedure is started.

Appropriate sedation or anesthesia is administrated. Local anesthesia is usually injected in the sterile area on the thigh. A small diagnostic flexible catheter is then inserted through the incision, directly into the femoral artery. Under fluoroscopic guidance, the catheter is advanced into the uterine artery.

Very small round particles (microspheres) are then injected through the catheter into the uterine artery. The flow of blood in the artery transports these tiny particles into the small blood vessels that supply blood to the fibroids. These particles occlude or block the flow of blood to these fibroids, and the fibroids shrink and die. Some of these fibroids are converted to scar tissue.

The embolization does not affect the normal muscles in the uterus because there are other blood vessels that supply the uterus. As a result, successful pregnancies have occurred after UAE. These pregnancies may be complicated by an increase in preterm or early deliveries.

61. What are the advantages of UAE?

First, UAE is regarded as an outpatient procedure, meaning the patient usually goes home after the procedure. Hospitalization, when needed, is usually for pain control only, and usually lasts about 24 hours.

The recovery period is much shorter than with the usual surgical treatment for fibroids. The patient is generally able to resume normal activities and return to work in about 7 to 10 days. (Surgery usually has a 4 to 6 week recovery time.)

The risk of significant complications after UAE is much less than with a myomectomy or hysterectomy.

UAE is generally regarded as the safest therapeutic option available to appropriate candidates.

UAE is generally regarded as the safest therapeutic option available to appropriate candidates.

62. What are the contraindications or limitations of UAE?

Pregnant females or those planning to become pregnant are not candidates for UAE. Women with cancer of the uterus, cervix, or ovary should not have this procedure. Undiagnosed abnormal uterine bleeding is a definite contraindication to UAE, as this may be a symptom of an undiagnosed cancer.

Patients with fibroids that are 20-weeks' size or greater are not good candidates for UAE. The reduction in size of such large fibroids still leaves a significant bulk after treatment.

63. What instructions are usually given to patients when they are discharged home after having UAE?

Upon discharge:

- Patients are given a prescription for pain medication with specific instructions on its use. They may also be given medications to treat nausea as well as medications to promote sleep with instructions to use them as needed.
- Patients are advised to refrain from any excessive physical activity for at least 2 weeks.
- Patients are given an appointment for follow-up evaluation with the interventional radiologist as well as the gynecologist.
- Finally, patients are given very strict and clear instructions to contact their doctors if any noticeable side effects (such as bleeding, severe pain, dizziness, or vomiting) occur.

PART SEVEN

Myomectomy

My gynecologist is recommending myomectomy.
Can you tell me more about this alternative
to hysterectomy?

What is a hysteroscopic-assisted myomectomy?

What is a resectoscope?

More . . .

64. My gynecologist is recommending myomectomy. Can you tell me more about this alternative to hysterectomy?

Myomectomy is a surgical procedure in which fibroids are removed individually, and it can be performed in one of several ways. The least invasive options are the vaginal procedures, which involve the use of specialized instruments: a **hysteroscope**, a resectoscope, or a laparoscope. Minimally invasive laparoscopic surgery, which involves a small keyhole incision, is another approach. Another option is an open **abdominal surgery**, or laparotomy.

The aim of a myomectomy is to remove individual fibroids as a way to preserve the uterus. Any of the surgeries can be tedious, depending on the number of fibroids that are present and where they are found in the uterus. You may also want to note that fibroids have been known to return in some women who have had myomectomies.

If you are planning to undergo one of the vaginal procedures, you will probably want to seek out an endoscopic surgeon who has performed many of the procedures. About 40,000 myomectomies are performed annually in the United States compared with 200,000 hysterectomies for uterine fibroids. Many women who choose myomectomy do so because they hope to become pregnant in the future. The National Uterine Fibroids Foundation (NUFF) suggests the procedure may also be helpful for women nearing menopause who, because of a decline in cycling ovarian hormones, probably wouldn't experience a fibroid resurgence.

Carolyn's comment:

After learning about all of my options for treatment, I chose to have a myomectomy because I still wanted to have the

Hysteroscope

A diagnostic procedure that uses a telescopic instrument to inspect the uterus.

Abdominal surgery

A surgical procedure performed through an incision similar to that of a cesarean section.

If you are planning to undergo one of the vaginal procedures, you will probably want to seek out an endoscopic surgeon who has performed many of the procedures.

possibility of becoming pregnant, and this procedure would ensure that the uterus was still viable for that. My surgery was very successful and without complication, although the size of the fibroid was a surprise; it was described as being like a football!

Kimberlee's comment:

My first surgery was a myomectomy, and I was terrified. I knew it was a major surgery, and I was concerned about how difficult the recovery would be. On my preop appointment, my doctor as a rule went over the entire procedure with me layer by layer. It was difficult to hear at the time, but in hindsight it was very reassuring. I was in the hospital for 3 days after the surgery and sitting up in a chair the day following my procedure. I was of course uncomfortable at first, but with taking short walks and sitting in chairs, the recovery went very fast.

65. What are the potential risks of the myomectomy surgery?

Abdominal myomectomy is a major surgery, whether it is done by laparotomy or laparoscopically. The potential risks are as follows:

- Pain
- Bleeding—The amount of blood lost during the surgery may require a transfusion.
- Development of blood clots—Clots usually occur in the lower extremities.
- Potential injury to internal organs, such as the bladder, intestines, and uterus.
- Infection
- Recurrence of fibroids—Studies suggest a recurrence rate of 26% within 5 years. The recurrence rate is greater when the surgery is done laparoscopically.

- Development of partial small bowel obstruction—
  This condition may occur from a few days to a few
  weeks after surgery.

Deborah's comment:

*My second myomectomy occurred on December 12, 2000,
at age 38. Fertility was still of paramount importance to
me and after conducting much research on the uterine
embolization procedure, which was considered experimental at the time, I opted to have another myomectomy.
Approximately 7 fibroids were removed (the largest being
6 cm) and my bladder was no longer under stress. I was
doing well until my wellness office visit with Dr. Greig in
Fall 2001, in which he told me the pelvic ultrasound report
indicated that I had innumerable myomas. I was devas-
tated to hear that news. I could not believe the fibroids
grew back so quickly after surgery.*

66. What is a hysteroscopic–assisted myomectomy?

Hysteroscopic myomectomy has been shown to be
effective in controlling the very heavy abnormal bleeding caused by submucosal fibroids. Hysteroscopic-
assisted myomectomy involves the aid of a slender,
lighted tubelike instrument. The device is inserted
through the vagina, so no incision is made in this procedure. It can be performed in an outpatient surgery
center. Miniature instruments are used as part of the
operation to remove fibroids (and/or uterine polyps
when they are present). If you are to undergo operative
hysteroscopic myomectomy, this method is used in the
removal of submucosal fibroids.

67. What is a laparoscopic myomectomy?

The laparoscope is an instrument used in minimally
invasive surgery. The technique is as follows.

A small quarter-inch incision is made just below the navel, and a special needle is gently inserted through this incision. This needle is attached to a special machine that is used to gradually pump air into the abdomen, resulting in the abdominal wall being pushed away from the internal organs (intestines, uterus, and liver).

Next, the laparoscope, which is a long pencil-like metal instrument, is inserted into the abdomen through the same incision. The laparoscope has a light at its far end, and a small video camera can be attached to its upper end. Once it is in place, live pictures are projected to television monitors stationed in the operating room.

The surgeon then makes additional small incisions near the pubic hair line; additional small surgical instruments are inserted through these incisions. The surgeon can proceed with the operation by looking directly at the television monitor.

Myomectomies or hysterectomies can be safely performed using this technique, depending on the size of the fibroids or uterus.

68. What is a resectoscope?

The resectoscope is actually a hysteroscope equipped with a special wire loop capable of emitting high electrical energy. This device is used to cut or resect growth such as submucosal fibroids.

The resectoscope is inserted through the vagina into the cervix, with a picture of the operative field being projected on a television screen. This procedure can also be used to remove uterine (**endometrial**) **polyps**. Like the conventional hysteroscopic procedure, a

Endometrial polyps

Small benign growths that protrude into the uterus.

resectoscopic myomectomy can be performed in an outpatient surgery center.

69. Does having a myomectomy mean I will need a cesarean section when I become pregnant?

The general rule is that a cesarean section is advisable if you have had significant surgical invasion of the wall of the uterus during a myomectomy. Most studies however tend to show a very low incidence of uterine rupture in pregnant women who have had prior myomectomy. It must be emphasized that rupture of the uterus can cause very serious complications for both the mother and the baby.

Kimberlee's comment:

My doctor delivered my son via a cesarean section. He wanted to deliver via cesarean to ensure there would be no complications from the previous surgery. I gave birth in 1998, and for the next 5 years I had no symptoms of fibroids.

PART EIGHT

Hysterectomy

My doctor has recommended a hysterectomy, but I understand there are pros and cons to the surgery. What should I know about the big picture?

How effective are less invasive alternatives?

When should I consider a hysterectomy?

More . . .

70. My doctor has recommended a hysterectomy, but I understand there are pros and cons to the surgery. What should I know about the big picture?

Despite concerns dating back 40 years that far too many women undergo hysterectomies, the procedure remains the most common nonobstetrical form of surgery performed on women in the United States today. Hysterectomy is surpassed only by cesarean section in the number of operations women undergo annually. Statistics from the Centers for Disease Control and Prevention (CDC) show that an estimated one in four women will have her uterus and very likely her ovaries removed by the time she reaches her 60th birthday. While the overall rate at which the surgery is performed has decreased significantly since the 1980s, rates vary further by age, region, and levels of education.

Not only are women more likely to undergo hysterectomies at a slightly younger age in some parts of the United States than in others, statistics also show that women with only a high school education are more likely to have a hysterectomy than those who attended college or completed more advanced degrees. The latter phenomenon suggests that women who are better educated are more likely to avail themselves of information about alternative procedures and to actively pursue those treatments. Nevertheless, statistics provide broad assessments, painting generalities that may have very little in common with your individual circumstances, and as such, that may not pertain to you. Hysterectomy is a surgery that has remained an inescapable fact of life for countless women in the United States regardless of social class, race, and level of education.

Hysterectomy is a surgery that has remained an inescapable fact of life for countless women in the United States regardless of social class, race, and level of education.

If you have a condition that has not been controlled by less invasive methods and your physician is recommending a hysterectomy, you will want to know as much as possible about the procedure. On the other hand, if you think the surgery has been recommended as your only choice and you would like to know about a less drastic alternative, then you will want to investigate your options, seek a second opinion, and find the best way to alleviate your medical problem by avoiding a major operation that requires weeks of recuperation.

Basically, the term *hysterectomy* refers to the removal of the uterus, which is also called the womb. Of course, depending on the diagnosis, other reproductive structures might also be removed to effectively treat a specific condition. In addition to the uterus, the procedure can include the cervix, the fallopian tubes, and the ovaries. You may have heard the term **total hysterectomy**, which on first blush seems to refer to the surgical removal of all reproductive tract structures. It actually refers to the removal of the uterus and cervix. The surgery that usually is performed for pelvic-area disease other than cancer is a **partial hysterectomy**—the removal of the pear-shaped uterus.

Total hysterectomy

The surgical removal of the uterus and cervix.

Partial hysterectomy

The surgical removal of the pear-shaped uterus, leaving the cervix in place.

Hysterectomy is a form of surgery that has its roots in a centuries-old past. Its very name recalls Greek origins: *bysterikos*, which refers to the womb, and *hystera*, the Greek word for hysteria. The term hysterectomy stems from the ancient notion that women were more likely than men to lose control emotionally and become hysterical. Removing the womb, the ancients believed, delivered women from the source of their madness. It took centuries for such ill-founded beliefs to fade.

Today, hysterectomy is one choice for the treatment of major reproductive system disorders, but it exists increasingly in an area of less invasive medical procedures, many involving groundbreaking technological innovations. Still, when medically warranted, a hysterectomy has helped to dramatically change lives that once were dominated by pain, bleeding, and disability.

Several key intellectual advances over the past 25 years have had an impact on hysterectomies. Newer, less radical alternatives have helped force a 20% decline in the number of hysterectomies performed annually in the United States. Also, there has been a keener understanding of the psychological impact that a hysterectomy can have—both good and bad—on women who undergo the surgery. For instance, when the procedure ends abnormal uterine bleeding, eliminates the further threat of cancer, or frees patients from a source of excruciating pain, then its psychological boost is said to be immeasurable. On the other hand, because the surgery ends the ability to reproduce, for those women who held hopes for bearing children, its impact can be psychologically difficult.

71. Why is a hysterectomy performed?

Several medical conditions have long been associated with hysterectomy:

- Uterine fibroids: As discussed throughout this book, these benign tumors can cause severe abnormal bleeding and extreme pain.
- Endometriosis: In this disorder, the uterine tissue inappropriately implants itself outside the uterus and throughout the pelvic area, triggering severe pain and irregular menstrual bleeding.

- **Uterine prolapse**: In this condition, the uterus (and in some instances the bladder as well) drops from its normal position and protrudes into the vagina.
- **Pelvic inflammatory disease (PID)**: This disorder results from overwhelming infections.
- Cancer: Cancer can affect any of the pelvic structures.

Certainly there are other conditions for which the surgery is performed, but the primary one in the United States is uterine fibroid tumors, growths that sometimes lead to such profuse bleeding that women must be treated in hospital emergency rooms. Cancer generally is perceived to be the strongest reason to perform the operation and is the condition for which there are the fewest alternative procedures.

72. What are the long-term side effects of hysterectomy? Are there ways I can avoid them or keep them at bay?

Although some women have reported long-term **depression**, sexual dysfunction, and fatigue following their surgeries, the most obvious long-term effects of a hysterectomy are an end to fertility, menstruation, and childbearing in women of reproductive age. The goal set by most physicians performing hysterectomies on patients of reproductive age is to leave the ovaries intact when at all possible, thus preserving hormone production.

Despite physicians' hopes of maintaining patients' capacity to produce hormones, there are cases when doing so is impossible. For example, when cancer is present, the ovaries must be removed. The same may hold true in certain instances of endometriosis when the ovaries are excessively overcome by endometrial

Hysterectomy

Uterine prolapse

Also known as pelvic relaxation, this condition occurs when the ligaments that hold the uterus and/or bladder in place loosen. Severe weakening may allow the organ(s) to protrude through the vagina.

Pelvic inflammatory disease (PID)

Acute or chronic inflammation of female pelvic structures (endometrium, uterine tubes, and pelvic peritoneum) due to infection (gonorrhea, chlamydia, and other organisms). If left untreated, PID can result in scarring and infertility.

Depression

A mental condition marked by sadness, inactivity, and an inability to think clearly. Depression is also characterized by feeling of dejection or hopelessness, and a significant increase or decrease in sleeping. In severe cases there may be suicidal tendencies.

implants and scarring, or in cases of pervasive pelvic inflammatory disease. Removing the ovaries (a surgical procedure known as **oophorectomy**) can trigger the immediate onset of menopause and its potent symptoms: hot flashes, night sweats, mood swings, vaginal dryness, and short-term memory loss, to name a few. Surgically induced menopause is sudden and dramatic. The long-term side effects of removing the ovaries can include an increased risk of osteoporosis (bone loss), heart disease, decreased muscle mass, a gradual change in the distribution of body fat, and a loss of libido (sexual drive).

It is possible to reduce the intensity of some of those side effects by replacing the estrogen that you are no longer able to produce on your own. Your doctor can write a prescription for estrogen replacement therapy. Estrogen replacement, however, is not without its own set of risks and may trigger a host of concerns that you will want to discuss with your healthcare provider. You definitely will want to know if taking estrogen is right for you.

Rigorous clinical trials have shown an increased risk for strokes and abnormal blood clotting, not only among women on estrogen therapy but also for those taking another type of hormone therapy in which pills containing both estrogen and progestin are prescribed. This type of hormone therapy, commonly called **hormone replacement therapy (HRT),** is prescribed to women who still have a uterus. For them, estrogen-only pills would greatly increase the risk of uterine cancer. These women still are not home free; HRT elevates the risk of breast cancer. Results from the Women's Health Initiative (WHI), a massive study of health concerns involving postmenopausal women, did

Oophorectomy

Removal of the ovaries. This can trigger the immediate onset of menopause and menopausal symptoms, including hot flashes, night sweats, mood swings, vaginal dryness, and short-term memory loss.

Hormone replacement therapy (HRT)

Medication containing one or more female hormones. HRT is most often used to treat symptoms of menopause, including hot flashes, vaginal dryness, mood swings, sleep disorders, and decreased sexual desire. Estrogen replacement therapy is a form of HRT that includes only the estrogen hormone.

not find an elevated breast cancer risk in women who had undergone a hysterectomy and who took estrogen-only pills.

The analysis of nearly 11,000 women who were randomly assigned to take either a daily estrogen pill or a placebo found that participants who took the hormone faced no greater danger of breast cancer than those taking dummy pills. However, WHI researchers found in a separate arm of their research that women on estrogen therapy had an elevated risk of deep vein thrombosis, a potentially fatal clotting condition in which a blood clot can travel through he bloodstream and lodge in a lung or cause a stroke. Smokers should be especially aware of the risks associated with abnormal clotting. If you want to take estrogen pills after your ovaries have been removed, then you will have to break your habit. It is important to discuss these matters thoroughly with your physician, especially if there are any issues suggesting that estrogen therapy could prove riskier than usual for you. Also, if you are around 50 years of age and nearing a natural menopause, you may not want to invite the risks inherent in taking estrogen pills and may choose to avoid hormone therapy altogether. Again, even this choice is something you will want to discuss with your doctor. Prevailing medical wisdom suggests a cautious approach to estrogen therapy, despite the news that estrogen-only pills do not increase the risk of breast cancer. Women should take the lowest dose to control hot flashes and other symptoms for the shortest time possible.

As ominous as the discussion has seemed so far, none of this is aimed at suggesting that estrogen replacement is a proposition entirely filled with risks. The therapy may have a long-term dividend, at least in one key respect: estrogen has the capacity to help prevent the development of osteoporosis, a disabling condition in which bones can easily fracture.

Meanwhile, the long-term side effects of hysterectomy are still being studied because they have raised serious research questions. Scientists are asking whether the surgery causes urinary incontinence in some women. Can a hysterectomy increase the likelihood of chronic constipation? Can diminished sexual response be a long-term side effect of the operation? While the answer is yes to all of these questions, none of the problems are pervasive among women who have had a hysterectomy. They are, however, common enough to have raised concern.

For example, regarding urinary incontinence, there have been mixed results from studies investigating hysterectomy's impact on bladder function. Some studies have found a link between the surgery and urinary incontinence, while others have not. Among those studies that have pinpointed a link, doctors say damage occurred to pelvic nerves during the operation or to pelvic support structures. Either way, bladder function was adversely affected. Surgical injury is not restricted to the most invasive form of hysterectomy. Urinary tract injuries have been known to occur with a minimally invasive hysterectomy in which the uterus is removed through the vagina. Researchers have been working on nerve-sparing surgical techniques as well as ways to avoid urinary tract injury.

Although not very common, another possible long-term side effect is slow-propulsion constipation, a disorder that also is known as slow-transit constipation. The American Society of Colon and Rectal Surgeons lists hysterectomy as one of many possible causes of this chronic condition and attributes the problem to localized damage to pelvic nerves sustained during surgery. Yet even with an established link between the chronic form of constipation and hysterectomy, doctors point to numerous other causes, which can include the use or abuse of certain medications, particularly opioid drugs, anticonvulsants, and calcium- or aluminum-containing antacids, among other medications. Such constipation also can occur as a consequence of diabetes and in certain anxiety disorders. Slow-propulsion constipation is treatable in many cases through simple dietary changes.

Finally, some women have reported diminished sexual responses as a post-hysterectomy side effect—something they say also diminishes their quality of life.

73. How effective are less invasive alternatives?

There are therapeutic options for many reproductive system disorders that once were treated exclusively by hysterectomy. Today, women have more options than they did just a decade ago. Conservative techniques and procedures can effectively treat reproductive organ problems without resorting to hysterectomy. With the exception of cancer, physicians begin by recommending alternative treatments to patients. If you are told that you need a hysterectomy for a noncancerous condition but are not first told of alternative therapies, then it may be wise to seek a second opinion. The American College of Obstetricians and Gynecologists, the leading professional organization of OB/GYN physicians, states in both its patient and physician education materials that "hysterectomy should be performed only for medical reasons, and only after alternative options have been discussed and explored with the patient."

Alternative treatments can be as simple as common pain relief medications, such as ibuprofen, naproxen, and even enteric-coated aspirin. Other medications, such as birth control pills, are also very familiar. Additional treatments, such as various forms of hormone-based medications, can be used for certain disorders to induce a pseudo-menopausal state. These drugs are administered over several months, allowing time for symptoms of your underlying condition to subside. In the best-case scenario, these medications can force the disorder into retreat.

Overall, the list of alternative treatments has grown substantially over the years and now includes many high-tech procedures. **Lasers** can be used against some conditions. Blood vessels that supply bothersome fibroids can be blocked with the infusion of tiny "microspheres" (see Question 60). By obstructing blood flow into the fibroids, the growths are forced to shrink. Fertility-sparing surgeries for several other types of reproductive system disorders (including fibroids) can provide relief from abnormal bleeding or pain while helping you avoid a hysterectomy.

Laser

A high-energy light source that emits a beam in a specified wavelength. A laser can quickly vaporize abnormalities with its heat.

Certainly, the aim here is not to give the impression that conservative procedures are completely free of risks and disappointments. Alternatives to hysterectomy come with their own set of drawbacks. Fertility-sparing surgeries may not be successful, and attempts to end excessive bleeding through drug therapy may not work. You as a patient may even become frustrated by the treatments when the results do not seem immediate. Still, when turning to alternative procedures, the goal is to maintain fertility and to put off—forever if possible—the need for a dramatically more invasive solution.

While on the subject of alternative procedures, you may find it noteworthy that the results of numerous studies have shown that alternative treatments tend to be less expensive, less debilitating, and less likely to cause a loss of productivity due to weeks spent recuperating. Recuperation after alternative procedures is significantly shorter compared with the 4 to 6 weeks spent in recuperation after a hysterectomy.

Alternative treatments tend to be less expensive, less debilitating, and less likely to cause a loss of productivity due to weeks spent recuperating.

74. Given the growing number of alternate procedures, could hysterectomy become passé?

Even in light of a 20% decline in the number of hysterectomies performed over the past quarter-century, which has been attributed to the increasing number of successful alternative treatments for female reproductive disorders, an estimated 650,000 to 675,000 women still undergo the operation annually in the United States (with at least 200,000 of these procedures due to uterine fibroids), according to data from the Centers for Disease Control and Prevention (CDC). Indeed, more hysterectomies are performed in the United States than in any other Western nation. A study by the Agency for Healthcare Research and Quality (AHRQ) found that 5 in every 1000 women in the United States undergo the operation each year compared with fewer than 3 in every 1000 in Great Britain and fewer than 2 in every 1000 in Norway. On the whole, European nations report substantially lower hysterectomy rates than the United Stares, a country where an estimated $5 billion in healthcare costs are spent on the surgery annually.

75. Are American physicians more likely to "believe" in hysterectomies?

Hysterectomy is neither a belief system nor a philosophy. It is a surgical procedure requiring a great deal of skill, performed by physicians who are specifically trained to treat conditions of the female reproductive system. But that does not mean all doctors are comfortable with the relatively high number of women who have the operations yearly in the United States. In a report produced by the U.S. Food and Drug Administration that examined alternatives to hysterectomy, Dr. Anthony Scialli (Georgetown University Medical Center, Washington, D.C.) said there are strong reasons to support the surgery in certain instances. In the report, Scialli is quoted as saying, "There are cases where hysterectomy is the only option. But I think we perform too many hysterectomies. It's a matter of American gynecologists being accustomed to performing a hysterectomy and American women being accustomed to getting one based on their mother or other female relative having one. The one thing in favor of a hysterectomy is that it works for abnormal bleeding—but it should be the last step, not the first step."

76. What are the different ways in which a hysterectomy is performed?

The surgery can be performed either through an abdominal incision or vaginally. Those are your choices. If you are to have the surgery, then you'll want to thoroughly discuss with your physician why a specific surgical method is being recommended. Your surgeon will examine you, evaluate your level of disease, and then recommend the method that will be most effective in the treatment of your condition. Abdominal surgeries generally are chosen for fibroids of relatively large size, certain cases involving endometriosis, and for any form of cancer (ovarian, **endometrial**, or cervical). Numerous studies have shown that for noncancerous conditions, doctors should strive for vaginal surgeries (removing the uterus through the vagina) when at all possible. There is more than one technique that can be employed to accomplish this task, which will be explained here.

Endometrial cancer

A malignancy that affects cells lining the uterus.

First, it is important to underscore that the way in which your operation is performed can have a bearing on the amount of time you spend recuperating. Abdominal surgeries (which are performed through an incision similar to that for a cesarean section) are associated with longer recovery periods and more manipulation of other abdominal structures during surgery (your intestines get jostled a bit); also there is a greater degree of postoperative pain. Recovery can take up to 6 weeks. The majority of hysterectomies performed in the United States are abdominal procedures.

The way in which your operation is performed can have a bearing on the amount of time you spend recuperating.

On the plus side, the abdominal operation allows your surgeon a keen view of the uterus and other reproductive organs and sufficient space to remove large fibroids, which sometimes can reach the size of a grapefruit or even larger. An abdominal hysterectomy, nevertheless, will leave a scar. With vaginal procedures, weeks are eliminated from the recovery period (the recovery takes about a month), and your bowel function returns sooner because there is far less interference with your intestines during surgery. Generally, the overall surgery is less painful. That said, the National Uterine Fibroids Foundation (NUFF), a nonprofit information clearinghouse based in Colorado, estimates that up to 144 million work hours are lost annually to recuperation from hysterectomies, regardless of how they are performed. Through its Web site, NUFF promotes awareness about the number of hysterectomies performed in the United States, especially for uterine fibroids, and underscores that women need to know about less invasive alternatives.

77. My physician is recommending a vaginal hysterectomy. What should I know about this procedure?

Vaginal hysterectomies are less debilitating than abdominal procedures. They can be performed in one of two ways: conventionally or with the aid of a laparoscope. In the conventional procedure, your surgeon makes a cut (called an incision) at the top of the vagina. Through this opening, the surgeon can cut and tie off ligaments and blood vessels. During this process, the fallopian tubes are also disconnected from the uterus, but left in place. The uterus is then freed and removed through the vagina.

A more advanced surgical technique involves the use of a laparoscope, an instrument that allows your physician to inspect abdominal organs through a tiny camera that is part of the device (see Question 46). The laparoscope is inserted through a small incision near the navel. This type of operation often is informally referred to as keyhole surgery, owing to the tiny incision through which instruments are inserted. The procedure also requires vaginal surgery and hence is known as a laparoscopic-assisted vaginal hysterectomy (LAVH).

About 10% of hysterectomies performed in the United States are laparoscopic-assisted. This form of surgery is considered to be far less traumatic, and the amount of time devoted to recovery is lessened as a result.

Vaginal hysterectomy

Type of surgery that removes the uterus through the vagina.

A study by the Agency for Healthcare Research and Quality (AHRQ) showed that in the 1990s the number of laparoscopic-assisted hysterectomies increased 30-fold, a trend that is strongly influencing how some surgeons are performing the operation now. However, the AHRQ also underscored that the abdominal hysterectomy remains the most common procedure in the United States, accounting for 63% of all hysterectomies. In France and Australia, by comparison, up to 50% of hysterectomy patients undergo vaginal operations.

78. What is the average age for hysterectomy? Does region play a role in hysterectomy?

Naturally, age varies among women undergoing hysterectomies each year in the United States, but government data show that approximately 55% of those who have the procedure are between 35 and 49 years of age. Within that group, women between the ages of 40 and 45 years are most likely to have the operation. Age has a strong relationship to hysterectomy because of the types of medical conditions that are most likely to occur during specific points in a woman's reproductive life.

For example, smaller proportions of women who undergo the procedure are older than 55 or younger than 30 years of age. Women in their mid-50s and older are more likely than younger women to have the surgery for some form of reproductive tract cancer, which may include ovarian, cervical, or uterine cancer.

Geographic region is an additional factor underlying the surgery's prevalence. For example, CDC statistics indicate that women who live in the South not only are more likely to undergo a hysterectomy than women who live in other parts of the country, they usually are younger than women elsewhere when they have the

Hysterectomy

procedure. Hysterectomy rates are lowest on the West Coast and in the Northeast, particularly in New York, which has the lowest rate of all 50 states and the District of Columbia. The average age of Southern women at the time of surgery is 41.6 years compared with 47.7 years for women in other parts of the country. Of course, there are no hard and fast rules regarding age and region. A woman living in California is as likely to undergo a hysterectomy at 35 years of age as is one living in Georgia, depending on each individual's diagnosis, symptoms, degree of discomfort, and personal choice. However, of the top 10 states reporting the highest rates of the operation, 7 are located in the Southeast.

79. When should I consider a hysterectomy?

A hysterectomy, generally, is not an operation that must be performed immediately unless the diagnosis is cancer, uterine hemorrhage, intractable pain, or an obstetrical emergency. Therefore, you have time to thoroughly discuss the operation with your physicians and even to ask whether there may still be a chance that an alternative to hysterectomy might better address your reproductive system disorder. If the answer to that question is no, and when symptoms have continued unabated despite earlier treatment through an alternative to hysterectomy (and the consensus opinion of your physicians is a recommendation of hysterectomy), then the surgery may be your best option. Again, the primary reasons for the surgery are cancer, obstetrical emergencies, uterine prolapse, excessive bleeding that leads to severe anemia and exhaustion, or intractable pain.

You have time to thoroughly discuss the operation with your physicians and even to ask whether there may still be a chance that an alternative to hysterectomy might better address your reproductive system disorder.

If you are not undergoing the surgery for a malignant condition, you may want to ask yourself some tough questions: What would the loss of a uterus, or possibly even both ovaries, mean to me? Do I want to take estrogen replacement therapy? Am I prepared to handle the psychological fallout from the operation, such as the thought of never being able to bear children (if you are of reproductive age)?

Of course, you may want to frame your questions in other ways: What new interests can I pursue once I am freed from excessive bleeding and pain? How much happier will I be when I am no longer worried about unpredictable bleeding?

Another thought to keep in mind if you are strongly considering the surgery is your time spent recuperating from it. Hysterectomy is considered major surgery, and at least a month or more is needed for recovery. Can you be away from work for 6 weeks, which is the standard amount of recovery time for an abdominal operation? Finally, you may want to be honest with yourself and ask whether you have tried every possible conservative approach before consenting to invasive surgery.

Kimberlee's comment:

In 2003, I began to feel some of the pain, and then later the heavy periods began to emerge. I began having the ultrasounds to determine the size and location of the tumors, and I knew that another procedure was in my future. Reluctant at first, I tried to hold off as long as I could, but by mid-2008 I was becoming anemic and I knew that I needed to take care of the problem. After careful consideration, we opted for a hysterectomy. I knew that this was going to greatly improve my quality of life and I would no longer have to deal with this very frightening and stressful disease. Also, I wanted to be sure that if I had to experience another procedure it would be the last. At 44, single, with a

10-year-old son, I was no longer interested in giving birth, and although I would consider a blended family, having babies was no longer desirable to me.

Deborah's comment:

I knew it was time to finally go through with a hysterectomy when my period came unexpectedly while vacationing in Europe in September 2008 and prevented me from participating on a paid tour to Peru and Bolivia in November 2008 at the eleventh hour. Since at age 46, fertility is no longer an issue for me and having a high quality of life is far more important, my uterus was finally removed on April 8, 2009. It was actually the size of a basketball and the equivalent of the size of a uterus belonging to a woman who is five months pregnant!

80. Is a hysterectomy covered by insurance?

Many insurers classify the surgery as elective unless it is being performed for cancer, an obstetrical emergency, or uterine hemorrhage. Some insurers also balk at covering a hysterectomy without the benefit of a second opinion. If this happens to you, it means that another physician will probably have to evaluate your case and arrive at the same conclusion before your health plan agrees to cover the surgery's expense. Additionally, for anyone who has recently signed on to a new health insurance plan, there may be a rule requiring a waiting period of at least 6 months before the operation is covered. Waiting may seem unfair, especially if you are experiencing symptoms that you and your physicians believe are best remedied by surgery. Some insurance companies, however, have taken a stance that too many of the operations are performed unnecessarily and that women should seek other, less expensive forms of care. These treatments may include taking pain relief medications or any one of several alternate procedures that do not involve surgery and hospitalization.

Of course, there is a counterpoint to this view: Insurance companies are committed to the bottom line. If there are strong medical reasons that surgery would be in your best interest, you should advocate strongly on your own behalf to receive it.

81. What should I do to prepare for a hysterectomy?

Certainly, you will have had a thorough pelvic examination during which your gynecologist manually inspected the uterus and other reproductive structures. You should also have had imaging tests, such as an ultrasound exam, to confirm your diagnosis. For your own peace of mind, you should make certain that you have been well informed about the procedure by your gynecologist and that surgery is warranted in your care. You also should avail yourself of any self-help information to ensure that you understand in lay terms exactly what is to occur surgically, that you know which structure(s) is being removed, and, if you are of reproductive age, that you understand you no longer will be fertile or able to menstruate.

If your insurance company requires a second opinion, then you will have the recommendation for a hysterectomy from more than one source. In addition, you probably will also want to make certain that you understand the actual procedure that has been recommended, the method in which the surgery will be performed, and how long you can expect to be recuperating from the surgery. Once these preliminaries are behind you, your doctor will order a series of laboratory tests, which will likely include screens of

If there are strong medical reasons that surgery would be in your best interest, you should advocate strongly on your own behalf to receive it.

Hysterectomy

blood and urine. All hysterectomies are performed in a hospital. They are not in-office procedures. Prior to your operation, you will meet with an anesthesiologist who will explain the type of medications that will be used. You will sign an **informed consent form** for the operation. This is a legal document that explains the purpose of the surgery and confirms that you have been told about the surgery's details as well as its potential risks and complications.

Informed consent form

A legal document that explains any invasive medical procedure, which must be read and signed by the patient in advance. Most forms describe the procedure and indicate that you have been informed of its risks and benefits.

82. Can a hysterectomy affect my sex life?

Some women report varying degrees of sexual dysfunction after a hysterectomy, while others report experiencing no side effects whatsoever. Instead, they say that their sex lives improved after hysterectomy because they were no longer inhibited by abnormal uterine bleeding or the excruciating discomfort caused by a large encumbering fibroid, endometriosis, or other pain-producing pelvic conditions. Severe pain brought on by reproductive system disorders can severely limit the quality of sexual relationships, making intercourse difficult. When the source of the pain is alleviated, sex can become more enjoyable.

Sexual function itself is multifaceted. It includes physiological, psychological, and complex emotional responses that involve feelings toward your partner, the surroundings in which the sexual encounter occurs, and various notions about the sexual act. Even the level of stress in your life comes into play. Stress can diminish sexual desire. Medical investigations have revealed post-hysterectomy difficulties ranging from loss of libido to problems with arousal to loss of orgasmic quality. Some of these factors have very little to do with whether you have a uterus—which is not to diminish the role of the uterus in female sexuality.

The uterus is believed to be involved in women's sexual response and contracts during orgasms. For some women, the absence of uterine contractions after a hysterectomy may affect her capacity to enjoy sex. This sense of loss can be a source of great anxiety. But keep in mind sexual response not only is highly variable from one person to another, it is—as noted earlier—very complex. Uterine contractions may not dominate the quality of intercourse for some women. For women who had a type of uterine fibroid known as a submucosal fibroid, the loss of uterine contractions may have occurred long before the hysterectomy because the growth tends to distort uterine shape and lessen the organ's ability to contract.

Virtually any kind of pelvic surgery, including hysterectomy, has the potential to affect the nerves and blood vessels that supply the reproductive system. If a hysterectomy is being strongly recommended and you have concerns about sexual dysfunction, it is very important to have an open discussion with your physician before your surgery to understand how this can be avoided. Sometimes just knowing that your physician is confident and cares about issues that are important to you can help bolster your spirits as you face major surgery. Also, if you have already had the operation and believe you may be experiencing sexual dysfunction related to your surgery, you should discuss that matter with a gynecologist. It cannot be stressed enough that because the potential exists for nerve and blood vessels to be adversely affected, this does not mean that you will be harmed in any way. That is why talking with your gynecologist is so important.

Just gathering a sense of what the surgery entails beforehand and knowing which structures will be removed can provide you with a stronger idea of what will happen long before you are wheeled into the surgical suite. Medical researchers have only begun to study the full range of complaints women have made about sexual dysfunction following a hysterectomy. They also have begun to better gauge which complaints are most frequently reported. Sometimes the issue may be depression, which can have an effect on your sexual response. If such is the case, then counseling and/or medication may address the problem.

Here is something else that you may want to keep in the forefront of your thoughts: When balanced against reports from women who say their sex lives improved after a hysterectomy, it is clear that sexual dysfunction is not a universal complaint among the vast number of women who have had the surgery. Among those who say their sex lives improved, many point to being free of abnormal bleeding and/or pain, which allowed spontaneity to again become part of their sex lives.

Nevertheless, there are additional concerns involving sexual matters that you will want to make note of if you are having the surgery. Whether your operation is vaginal or abdominal, you will be advised against sexual intercourse for a few weeks after the procedure. Of course, this recommendation for temporary abstinence is for several reasons. Your doctor's chief concern is lowering your risk for infection. In addition, your healthcare provider will want to ensure that you give your pelvic area enough time to heal properly following the trauma of surgery and the loss of structures that once filled the space. While some women have remarked that they had resumed sexual activity with vigor and enthusiasm after the few weeks of abstinence following their operations, others report discomfort with intercourse. In some patients, the operation can result in scar tissue or even a slight shortening of the vaginal passageway.

If your ovaries are removed, your hormone levels are no longer what they used to be, so your libido may diminish and you may have additional problems with lubrication and vaginal dryness. These issues are not insurmountable; hormones can be prescribed to counteract issues with libido. The medications also can help enhance lubrication and combat vaginal dryness.

As for a shortened vagina, it can be stretched with repeated attempts at intercourse. The vagina is extraordinarily elastic, a fact that you are probably already well aware of if you have ever had a baby. The take-home message here is simple: You can regain a satisfying sex life after a hysterectomy. For some women, the transition from their preoperative sex lives to the ones after the operation is seamless. In fact, they remark that with the alleviation of problems with chronic bleeding and pain, sex was a welcome alternative. For others, achieving a healthy sex life after hysterectomy may require some effort. But if you and your partner are willing to work through the problem period, it is likely that you will be able to have a healthy sex life after your surgery.

83. Hysterectomy seems to be as much a political issue as it is a medical one. Why are women's health groups so concerned about the surgery?

Hysterectomy has generated intense concern among women's health advocacy groups for nearly half a century and usually for the very obvious reason that it is a major health intervention that hundreds of thousands of women face each year. Concerns about hysterectomy and its necessity are no longer just the turf of women's health groups but also have become a focus of health insurers, physicians, and major medical organizations. Virtually all of them recommend that women first try alternate procedures before agreeing to a hysterectomy when at all possible.

Women's health advocacy groups have long had a very specific aim: to help women make informed decisions about the operation and to spread the word about alternatives to the surgery. It would be both a disservice and a mistake to define members of these groups as hotheaded militants with political axes to grind. The groups are varied and cut across a wide spectrum of focus and influence. Yes, many women's health advocacy groups have been strongly motivated by the sheer number of hysterectomies performed annually in the United States. Yes, they have openly stated that many, if not most, of the operations might be avoidable, and their concern stems from the vast number of hysterectomies that are performed as elective procedures. Indeed, many believe that if women were better informed about alternatives, perhaps there would be fewer hysterectomies. But bear in mind that it was activism that first helped awaken the public—and the medical community—to the surgery's extreme overuse a generation ago. From these groups' grassroots efforts, today other issues, such as calling attention to the types of subtle post-hysterectomy side effects that may take years or even decades to manifest, have become yet another rallying point.

Years ago, women took aim against what they felt was an insensitive medical community, which they believed viewed the female reproductive system as a useless group of organs once women had finished childbearing or had reached a certain age. Sherrill Selman, author of the book *Hormone Heresy*, wrote in an essay entitled "Hysterectomy Heresy" that women faced a formidable medical community in the early 1970s. Many doctors felt hysterectomy should be the norm. "The overwhelming conclusion regarding whether every woman who is finished with childbearing should have a hysterectomy was summed up by gynecologists Ralph W. White," Sellman reported in a retrospective of the 1971 meeting of the American College of Obstetricians and Gynecologists. She continued, "He expressed the members' prevailing attitude of respect for the female womb by proclaiming, 'It's a useless, bleeding, symptom-producing, potential cancer-bearing organ.'"

In the 21st century, the Internet has helped women's health organizations evolve beyond the bitter issues of the 1960s and 1970s. Women are being invited into online support and discussion groups in which any issue is open to debate. Post-hysterectomy sexual response, incontinence, depression, fatigue, relationship issues, weight gain—you name it—are all being discussed online. Chat formats on numerous Web sites have allowed women facing hysterectomy to discuss their fears with those who have already undergone the surgery.

Of course, you may ask what these organizations are like. Some groups have broad memberships that are open to women with any type of condition that can lead to a hysterectomy. Other groups are more narrowly focused and deal with a single medical condition that can result in the surgery. For instance, the group may focus its interests on endometriosis, uterine fibroids, or gynecological cancers. While such organizations have an interest in hysterectomy, they also are focused on conveying information about the medical conditions to which they are devoted.

Finally, a group may be quite general in its aim, with its membership composed of women who underwent or who are considering the surgery for any number of reasons. These groups are not concerned about controversies surrounding the surgery, but the way in which women are coping pre- and post-hysterectomy. A prime example of the latter is a group that calls itself Hyster-Sisters.com, a Denton, Texas, online organization that offers support groups via its Web site. This site allows women to discuss their fears and concerns regarding hysterectomy and other, less invasive alternatives. In its published mission statement, the group defines itself as "neither anti-hysterectomy nor pro-hysterectomy," which is proof that women's health groups can be concerned about the surgery without taking a political stance. The group does not avoid controversial subjects. Topics such as sexual dysfunction and troubles women have experienced with estrogen replacement therapy after the operation are open to discussion by Web site visitors.

Certainly, this is not to say that women's groups have mellowed and have lost the fire that fist helped them draw attention to the surgery and its aftereffects. Groups such as the HERS Foundation (Hysterectomy Education Resources and Services), based in suburban Philadelphia, take a far stronger position against the surgery and urge women through their Web sites and national conferences to avoid hysterectomies when at all possible. The HERS Foundation collects data on post-hysterectomy side effects through polling that it conducts. The data are maintained on the foundation's Web site.

For nearly a decade, the HERS Foundation sought information on the most common side effects from the surgery by polling women about their experiences. The group noted "personality change" as the number one long-term side effect reported by most women who had undergone a hysterectomy and who responded to the foundation's questionnaire. HERS defines its mission as providing information about "alternatives to, and consequences of, hysterectomy," and urges women to actively seek alternatives to the surgery. The foundation also has called on women to protest unwarranted hysterectomies.

The HERS Foundation's battle cry, which would have been considered radical a generation ago, increasingly has found reinforcement in mainstream medicine, which independently has demonstrated through rigorous scientific research that many claims from advocates have been right on target. In a study published in the *Journal of Obstetrics and Gynecology*, Dr. Michael Broder (a medical researcher at the University of Southern California) reported that 70% of the surgeries were probably recommended inappropriately and that women who were told they needed to have a hysterectomy could have fared better without the operation. Dr. Broder's study of 500 women who had undergone hysterectomies for nonemergencies also indicated that many of the patients had been inadequately evaluated for the surgery.

In that same vein, the National Uterine Fibroids Foundation (NUFF) has sounded an alarm about a range of problems associated with hysterectomies, from the number of procedures performed annually to the surgery's high-flying costs. The foundation devotes its energies to raising awareness about the high rate of hysterectomies performed for uterine fibroids and maintains a database of statistics about the surgery. It collects information from a variety of sources, such as the Centers for Disease Control and Prevention and the American College of Obstetricians and Gynecologists.

NUFF notes that for every 10,000 hysterectomies performed each year in the United States, 11 women die. A total of about 660 deaths a year are attributable to hysterectomy complications, according to the foundation. Among the more than 600,000 hysterectomies performed annually, 60% of patients have their ovaries removed, and more than $5 billion is spent on hormone replacement therapy alone. An additional $5 billion is spent for the surgery itself. Alarms from the NUFF and similar groups have not gone unheard. Some doctors inform their patients about the groups as a source of education.

Advocacy groups and mainstream medicine have found common ground in another area of concern: the need for a greater emphasis on research into new and better methods of treating female reproductive system disorders. Dr. Donna Shoupe (Women's and Children's Hospital in Los Angeles) was among the first physicians to question the wisdom of routinely removing the ovaries of women 45 years of age and older during hysterectomies, a practice that was very common as recently as the 1990s (and has yet to fully disappear).

Bilateral oophorectomy

Surgical removal of both ovaries.

Bilateral oophorectomies (surgical removal of both ovaries) were being performed along with the removal of the uterus based on the belief that women were more likely to develop ovarian cancer as they aged. Removing the ovaries, doctors thought, would reduce the cancer risks. But studies increasingly demonstrate that the ovaries still produce hormones in older women. The new discoveries are flying in the face of conventional wisdom, which generally considered the two glands as having virtually no function after menopause. Some studies now suggest the ovaries play a role well into the later years of life, producing hormones such as testosterone and minute amounts of estrogen for up to 10 years past menopause.

Many in the women's health advocacy community had long opposed the routine removal of the ovaries in women undergoing hysterectomies. Oophorectomies create an instant need for hormone replacement therapy, a treatment that has proven to be problematic in some women. Often, healthcare providers must work with them to find the formulation that is most helpful. In addition, routine oophorectomies also overlooked the role that the ovaries play in postmenopausal women.

84. Are there any positive factors related to hysterectomy?

Hysterectomy has many positives. In countless instances, hysterectomies have rescued women from life-threatening conditions. For those who have been treated for cancer, there is the relief of knowing that the cancer has been removed and a major step has been taken toward restoring health. There also is a feeling of relief among women whose lives were dominated by excessive blood loss, which led to anemia and its accompanying fatigue. And, there is a sense of relief from the intractable pain produced by endometriosis, large fibroids, or any other reproductive organ abnormality. Some women have even said their surgeries afforded them newfound freedom because their

In countless instances, hysterectomies have rescued women from life-threatening conditions.

lives were no longer limited by a chronic medical condition. To reiterate, though, hysterectomy generally is necessary only for disorders that are life-threatening, such as cancer, an obstetrical emergency, excessive bleeding, or severe uterine prolapse. For any other reason, the surgery is elective.

85. I have several uterine fibroids. Does that mean I need a hysterectomy?

No, it doesn't necessarily mean that a hysterectomy is the right option for you. Hysterectomy is an appropriate option for some women with extremely problematic fibroid tumors, but certainly not all. As mentioned earlier, many women live with fibroids and never experience symptoms. A procedure known as myomectomy, which is discussed in greater detail in Part 6, is a form of surgery that allows your doctor to remove individual fibroids while preserving the uterus and the capability to become pregnant. However, when a uterus is riddled with many fibroids, it may be virtually impossible to remove each fibroid individually and preserve the integrity of the uterus. In such an instance, especially when bleeding is prolonged and profuse and other treatments have failed, a hysterectomy might be the best choice. Still, it cannot be repeated enough: Before resorting to invasive surgery, your doctor will likely offer more than one alternate procedure in an attempt to address your problem conservatively.

Before resorting to invasive surgery, your doctor will likely offer more than one alternate procedure in an attempt to address your problem conservatively.

86. Please explain myolysis and cryomyolysis. These two alternates to hysterectomy sound very similar. How do they differ? Can they preserve fertility?

Unfortunately, neither of these treatments preserves fertility, and they are not widely offered to patients.

Both are geared toward eliminating troublesome fibroids that may be a source of excessive bleeding. While the two treatments are aimed at destroying uterine fibroids, they go about it in different ways. Both procedures are performed laparoscopically.

Myolysis is believed to work best on smaller fibroids and is not recommended for those that may have grown to the size of a cantaloupe. Treatment through myolysis allows your doctor to eliminate the fibroids' blood supply by using a laser or electrical current to cauterize (burn) the blood vessels feeding the growths. The technique usually is recommended to those who are not planning to have children, as serious complications of pregnancy have been known to occur among women who have been treated with this technique. Theoretically, once the blood supply to the fibroid has been eliminated, the growth then shrivels and dies. However, there have been no long-term studies on myolysis.

Cryomyolysis is very similar except that it uses a super-cooled probe to freeze the fibroids, which causes the growths to wither and die. A benefit is that it helps to prevent invasive surgery and removal of the uterus. Both procedures take about an hour to perform, and patients do not have to be hospitalized. After either procedure, patients have reported abdominal pain and cramping. Their discomfort can be treated with mild painkillers. Recuperation requires a few days compared with 6 weeks for a hysterectomy.

87. What is endometrial ablation, and is it useful in the treatment of fibroids?

When heavy abnormal uterine bleeding is the chief problem, **endometrial ablation** may be a very effective

---

Hysterectomy

Myolysis

A surgical procedure in which the blood supply to fibroids is halted, causing them to shrink and die.

Cryomyolysis

A surgical method that involves freezing fibroids, which forces them to shrink.

Endometrial ablation

An outpatient procedure that may involve using a laser to eliminate the cells lining the uterus. The procedure may make conception possible.

measure in women who do not wish to become pregnant in the future.

The object of this procedure is to destroy or alter the lining of the uterine cavity by applying heat or thermal energy, with the aid of the hysteroscope. Two of the more frequently used methods are laser ablation and hydrothermal ablation.

In some patients, endometrial ablation is effective in treating the abnormal uterine bleeding caused by submucosal fibroids.

In some patients, endometrial ablation is effective in treating the abnormal uterine bleeding caused by submucosal fibroids.

88. Does hormone replacement therapy have any effect on fibroids in menopausal women?

Some studies suggest that menopausal women who take hormone replacement medications are more likely to have abnormal bleeding. The hormonal replacement may cause an increase in the size of the fibroid.

89. My insurance company will not cover my hysterectomy until I have had a second opinion. Will my gynecologist feel insulted if I go to another doctor?

Insurance companies are in the business of earning profits. One way to ensure that they do so is to make certain that patients receive effective procedures at the lowest possible cost. Surgeries of all kinds are notoriously expensive and your insurer probably will want you to avoid an operation if at all possible—and that is not because the company loves you. Insurance companies want to keep the millions of dollars they have charged their customers for premiums. They do not want to spend the cash on expensive medical interventions.

For your peace of mind, you should actively seek the opinion of another physician to make certain the first doctor's recommendation for surgery is indisputable. Second opinions are important when major surgery is planned, regardless of the reason for the operation. Hysterectomy is just one of many procedures for which an insurer may demand a second opinion. In fairness to insurance companies, many are recommending evaluations by a disinterested second party because the companies have found some surgeries and diagnostic tests are performed unnecessarily and that patients may be better served by a less expensive procedure.

Second opinions are important when major surgery is planned, regardless of the reason for the operation.

Most insurers will pay for the cost of a second opinion, as will Medicare. In many states, Medicaid also will cover the cost. However, if your insurer is demanding a second opinion but will not cover the expense, you still may consider handling the cost yourself because of the value you will gain by having a second physician review your chart and tests. In instances when an insurer will not pay for the second opinion, it is also possible for you to appeal the refusal. Given that the insurance company demanded the second evaluation, you can make a case to the administrators of your health insurance plan.

While all of this may seem harassing at a time when you may not be feeling your best physically, bear in mind that a second opinion helps you more than it helps the insurance company. Hysterectomy can have a profound psychological impact on some women. As with any form of surgery, hysterectomy can produce anxiety, but it also causes postoperative pain and may even bring about menopause at an early age. Therefore, you will want to be certain that the procedure is warranted and necessary. You do not want to be misled into an operation that is irreversible.

Hysterectomy

Finally, you may even want to start a journal that will help you understand where you have been in your journey and whether you are comfortable with the prospect of having your uterus and possibly other reproductive structures removed, no matter what your age. Keep in mind that a hysterectomy can have a different effect based on how it is performed. For example, if your ovaries are left intact, you will continue to produce your natural flow of hormones. If you are being treated for a condition other than cancer and you have been told that your ovaries should be removed, you certainly will want a second opinion to fully understand the need for the more radical procedure.

Physicians are not insulted when their patients seek second opinions. They are accustomed to their patients going elsewhere for an additional opinion. Your doctor also is well aware that insurers often ask for second opinions, and many welcome an evaluation that will likely corroborate their medical judgment. Conscientious physicians welcome second opinions and encourage their patients to seek them. Your physician probably has given dozens of second opinions involving the recommendations of other physicians and is familiar with the need to offer an evaluation on another physicians' cases.

It's easy to say that you have seen your gynecologist for years and fully trust his or her medical judgment, but even in instances where there is a strong bond between doctor and patient, you owe yourself the peace of mind of knowing your doctor's diagnosis has been corroborated by another expert.

Also, it is important to note that standards mandating surgery can differ from one region of the country to another, from one hospital to the next, and even from one physician to another. With that in mind, it again is in your best interest to seek a second opinion. With respect to elective procedures (and a hysterectomy is one of them), you are the final arbiter on whether surgery is best in your case; you determine whether the pain associated with an invasive surgery is worth the time, money, and temporary physical discomfort. The most effective way to make this decision is by listening to what more than one doctor has to say. Every patient who is scheduled to have a hysterectomy or any major surgery should be encouraged by her physician to get a second opinion.

90. Can I seek a second opinion even if my insurance company has not requested one?

Yes, you can seek a second opinion for the reasons mentioned in Question 89. But this is definitely an instance in which an insurer would be least likely to cover the second opinion cost. Even when the insurer is not making the request, some women want second opinions about a recommendation of hysterectomy. A second opinion can offer the patient peace of mind for several reasons. A second doctor's evaluation may introduce the patient to a new alternative that her physician may not have offered or did not feel confident performing.

In the first few years when uterine artery embolization (UAE) became available, few doctors felt confident performing the procedure, and many others did not refer patients to physicians who were well trained in the technique. Doctors now are finding that UAE is becoming an important option that helps women avoid a hysterectomy.

On the other hand, a second opinion also can confirm that a hysterectomy is the best solution after what may have been a long and frustrating series of alternate treatments that proved futile. As discussed in Question 48, in instances when multiple fibroids have obstructed the uterus growing within its cavity and between its walls, procedures that attempt to remove the fibroids alone may not be possible. When the patient is suffering significant pain and excessive bleeding is causing severe anemia, a hysterectomy may be the best way to achieve relief. The surgery eliminates the source of pain and permanently stops the blood loss.

91. How do I get a second opinion?

Getting a second opinion may require some effort on your part. Your gynecologist can provide a recommendation. But it is probably wise to seek an opinion outside of your physician's own office, especially if your doctor is part of a group practice with other gynecologists. It is likely that they have discussed your case and already share a similar opinion on how it should be handled.

Ideally, it is best to seek a second opinion at a major teaching hospital (which is an institution where medical students, interns, and residents are trained). There you will find expert physicians on staff who would be willing to evaluate your case. Another way of finding a physician is to ask friends or family members, especially women who have had a medical problem similar to your own. If that route is not feasible, you can contact the local medical societies in your area or go online to the Web site of the American College of Obstetricians and Gynecologists (www.acorg.org), which maintains a database of member physicians throughout the United States. You may also elect to ask your family physician to refer you to another doctor for a second opinion.

92. What if the second opinion differs from the first?

You are an active participant in your health care, and when two doctors render completely different opinions, it is not a time for you to shy away in confusion. You should ask both physicians how they reached their conclusions, and why each has such divergent recommendations. You may also want to seek a third opinion. A third opinion that corroborates one of the first two may provide guidance on which path would be the best for you to take.

93. What medical information do I give the second gynecologist?

All of the medical information that has been gathered in your case is relevant for a second opinion. That information includes your medical records, ultrasound images, medication history, the outcome of previous alternative procedures, and your own oral history of your pain and/or abnormal bleeding. You can request as many opinions as you wish. As mentioned in the previous answer, two differing opinions can seem confusing, leaving the patient uncertain as to which physician is offering the best medical judgment in her case. When patients become their own health advocates, they actively seek answers to their questions.

A third opinion that corroborates one of the first two may provide guidance on which path would be the best for you to take.

94. What preparation do I need prior to my scheduled hysterectomy?

Before you undergo any major surgery (including hysterectomy), there are several important preparatory steps that must be taken:

1. Your doctor will thoroughly review your medical history and your physical examination.

2. The planned surgical procedure should be explained in detail to you in simple language, and all your questions should be fully answered.

3. Based on your age and medical history, there are certain laboratory evaluations that must be done. These may include:
   - A complete blood count to ensure that you have enough blood in your system to safely withstand a major operation.
   - Coagulation studies to indicate whether your blood clots normally and to help establish that you have no abnormal bleeding tendencies.

4. An electrocardiogram (EKG) may be performed to evaluate the status of your heart. This test is usually dictated by your age (45 years or older) and your medical history.

5. A chest X-ray is performed based on your age and medical history.

6. Medical clearance from your internist or primary care physician may be indicated. This also may depend on your age and medical history. If you have any significant medical problems such as heart disease, diabetes, or lung disease, a medical clearance may be requested by your gynecologist prior to surgery.

7. Finally, you will always be instructed to have NOTHING to eat or drink for at least 8 hours before the scheduled time for your surgery.

Authorization for your hospitalization and surgery should have been obtained from your medical insurance company. This is important, so that you will fully understand what your financial obligations are to the hospital as well as your doctor.

95. What may I expect to happen when I arrive at the hospital for my hysterectomy?

The procedures may be slightly different with each hospital. In general, you will go first to the admission department of the hospital where your insurance information and ability to pay for your hospital stay will be verified. From there you will be taken to the preoperative area, which is usually on the same floor as the surgical or operating rooms.

In the preoperative area, you will be asked to state your doctor's name and the proposed surgical procedure you will be undergoing. You will then be asked to sign a consent form, which ensures that the hospital and your doctor have your legal and informed permission to perform the surgery.

The staff at the hospital will identify themselves to you and will explain what their respective duties are. You will then be asked, in an appropriately private location, to change into a hospital gown furnished by the staff. Next, the anesthesiologist usually introduces himself or herself to you and fully explains what type of anesthesia will be used. Your questions and concerns about the anesthesia should be discussed at this time. Your surgeon will be present at this time and will be available for any questions that may arise.

The anesthesiologist will then start an intravenous line (IV) in one of your arms. You may receive some preoperative antibiotics intravenously at this point.

You will then be transported, usually in a gurney (mobile bed) to the operating room. Attending to you in the operating room will be your doctor, an assistant surgeon (if needed), the anesthesiologist, and at least two nurses. You will then be placed on the operating table, which may resemble a narrow bedlike structure.

At this point, a number of monitoring devices will be attached, painlessly, to you. These generally include:

- A blood pressure cuff,
- A pulse oximeter, which measures the amount of oxygen you are utilizing, and
- A cardiac monitor to constantly evaluate the activity of your heart.

The anesthesiologist will then administer medication intravenously to put you to sleep and will inform the surgical team when you have been adequately anesthetized.

An indwelling catheter (Foley catheter) will then be inserted through your urethra into the bladder. This catheter will be left in place throughout the surgical procedure for three basic reasons:

1. To keep the bladder deflated (empty), thereby reducing the risk of surgical injury to the bladder
2. To keep the bladder as small as possible to prevent blocking the surgeon's view during the operation
3. To indicate to the surgical team, through the constant draining of urine, how well your kidneys are functioning during the operation

The area on your body, through which the surgery will be performed (i.e., the abdomen and/or the vagina), will then be meticulously washed with special cleaning solutions in order to achieve a sterile surgical field.

The surgeon, dressed in sterile surgical gown and gloves, will then place sterile drapes over the proposed surgical area. Then the surgical procedure will begin.

96. What are the potential risks or side effects of a myomectomy or hysterectomy?

The primary surgical risks include:

1. Pain: To prevent pain, you will be given adequate anesthesia during the operation, and postoperatively you will be placed on pain medication as the need dictates.

2. Infection: Two very important steps are essential during this type of surgery:
   ○ Observation of sterile techniques
   ○ Administration of preoperative preventative antibiotics (these may at times also be administered during the operation)

3. Blood clots: Clots are a very serious potential risk. The surgeon will place special compression stockings on both lower extremities during and after surgery. In patients who, because of their medical history, are at increased risk for developing blood clots (thromboembolism), special blood-thinning medication (heparin) may also be administered.

4. Injury to internal organs: This is prevented by:
   ○ Keeping the bladder drained and empty during surgery
   ○ Packing the intestines away from the immediate surgical field with sterile towels
   ○ The surgeon's paying very strict attention to the various anatomical structures that he or she encounters

5. Bleeding or hemorrhage: The surgeon's skill and expertise will be used to identify the vascular structures,

and he or she will ligate (tie), occlude (clamp), or cauterize the blood vessels as the need dictates.

97. What can I expect after I am discharged home from the hospital?

Prior to your discharge from the hospital, you will be given very specific instructions about:

- Rest
- Activity
- Medications
- Potential developments such as fever, increased pain, and bleeding (You will be instructed to call your doctor immediately should any of these symptoms occur.)

You will also be given an appointment to see your doctor after your discharge from the hospital (usually in 1 to 2 weeks). The discharge instructions are the joint responsibility of your doctor as well as the nursing staff at the hospital.

Carolyn's comment:

Even during my first few days of recovery, I felt better. I felt more like my normal self. I was ready to resume all normal activity after about 4 weeks, including exercise, and by week 6, I got my doctor's approval to do so. It is a relief to know that the fibroid is gone now; I hadn't realized how much it had affected me all this time. A thin line of a scar is a small price to pay for how much better I feel now.

98. What shall I do about the disability forms that are required by my job as well as by the state?

These papers are usually completed and signed by your doctor. A small fee may be charged for this service.

Some employers require a signed medical release or return to work form. Such forms are also provided by your doctor.

99. What happens to the organs or tumors that are surgically removed by my doctor?

All organs, tumors, or tissue that are removed are labeled appropriately and sent to the pathology department at the respective hospitals. The pathologist meticulously examines the organs and tumors, microscopically, and then gives a final definitive diagnosis. Your doctor will then inform you of the final diagnosis and will tell you if any additional treatment is needed. You may also request copies of your medical records from your doctor as well as from the hospital. These copies will usually be supplied after you have signed a release of records form.

100. Will my medical insurance cover all the various therapeutic options?

You should contact your insurance company as soon as the method of treatment has been selected. Some insurance carriers may cover all or part of the expenses. Other carriers may not cover some procedures. Usually, your doctor's office will assist you in obtaining this information as well as getting the necessary authorization for treatment from the insurance company. You should be aware that, unless other arrangements are made, you will ultimately be held directly responsible for all the medical expenses incurred.

Specific Recommendations About Fibroids

The American College of Obstetricians and Gynecologists (ACOG) has issued the following recommendations:

1. Hysterectomy provides a definitive cure in women with symptomatic fibroids.

2. Abdominal myomectomy is a safe and effective option in women who wish to retain their uterus.

3. Women who undergo myomectomy should be counseled about the increased risk of recurrence of the fibroids.

4. The use of GnRH agonists (e.g., Lupron) is beneficial if one plans to shrink the fibroids and to decrease the rate of uterine bleeding.

5. The side effects and the cost of medication (e.g., Lupron) must be discussed in detail.

6. Hysteroscopic myomectomy is effective in controlling heavy menstrual bleeding in women with submucosal fibroids.

7. All therapeutic options should be fully discussed, even if the patient is postmenopausal.

Resources

American Society for Reproductive Medicine
Fibroid Special Interest Group
1209 Montgomery Highway
Birmingham, AL 35216-2809
Phone: (205) 978-5000
Web site: www.asrm.org
E-mail: asrm@asrm.org

The Fibroid Foundation
31 Pleasant Street
Medford, MA 02155
Web site: www.fibroidfoundation.org

Hope for Fibroids
Web site: www.hopeforfibroids.org
E-mail: hope@hopeforfibroids.org

National Uterine Fibroids Foundation
PO Box 9688
Colorado Springs, CO 80932-0688
Phone: (800) 874-7247
Web site: www.nuff.org
E-mail: info@nuff.org

Glossary

Abdominal surgery: A surgical procedure performed through an incision similar to that of a cesarean section.

Abnormal uterine bleeding: A disorder caused by any one of several underlying reproductive system conditions; characterized by excessive bleeding and/or blood clots that may lead to anemia.

Adenomyosis: A very painful condition characterized by the infiltration of glandular tissue from the lining of the uterus into the muscular portion of the uterine walls.

Adhesions: Fibrous bands of tissue that abnormally cling to nearby structures. They may cause major structures (e.g., ovary, outer walls of the uterus and bladder) to become stuck together. The condition produces extraordinary pain.

Anemia: A disorder in which there is a low red blood cell count so the red blood cells carry less oxygen. Anemia can result in fatigue and exhaustion

and if left untreated, may be life-threatening.

Anovulatory: Menstrual periods in which an egg is not produced.

Atypia: A term pathologists use to describe abnormal cells.

Bilateral oophorectomy: Surgical removal of both ovaries.

Bimanual examination: A type of investigation used for diagnosis, in which the physician places two lubricated gloved fingers into the vagina and pushes upward while also pressing down with the other hand on the outside of the lower abdomen. This action allows the gynecologist to feel any growths in the uterus or on the ovaries.

Biopsy: A surgical procedure in which a tiny sample of tissue is removed so that the cells can be viewed under a microscope and analyzed.

Birth control medications: Hormone-based drugs used primarily to prevent conception. Also used as treatments for fibroids and other reproductive system disorders.

Cancer: Any malignant development caused by abnormal and uncontrolled growth of cells. Some cancers grow rapidly and invade surrounding tissues and organs; others are more indolent and grow slowly.

Cervical dysplasia: The abnormal growth of cells on the surface of the cervix.

Cervical intraepithelial neoplasia (CIN): A precancerous condition caused by an abnormal growth of cells on the surface of the cervix. These cells can linger for long periods in a precancerous state before becoming invasive cancer.

Cervical polyps: Tiny growths that protrude inside the uterus and may be a source of abnormal bleeding.

Cervix: The neck at the lower end of the uterus. It connects the uterus to the vagina. The cervix dilates during labor to allow the birth of a baby.

Complex hyperplasia: A term used by pathologists to define an overgrowth of cells in the uterus in which the proliferation is so excessive that the structure of the uterus itself has changed. Microscopically, the infinitesimal glands of the endometrium can be seen crowding one another. The endometrium's stroma cells also exhibit marked proliferation.

Cryomyolysis: A surgical method that involves freezing fibroids, which forces them to shrink.

Depression: A mental condition marked by sadness, inactivity, and an inability to think clearly. Depression is also characterized by feeling of dejection or hopelessness, and a significant increase or decrease in sleeping. In severe cases there may be suicidal tendencies.

Dermatopontin: A protein made by the body to prevent cells from straying into aberrant patterns of growth. Researchers have associated low levels of the protein with the development of fibroid tumors.

Dilation and curettage (D&C): A diagnostic procedure performed when the woman is under general anesthesia or an epidural. The cervix is dilated and then the uterus is scraped with a spoon-shaped instrument called a curette. The resulting tissue specimen is sent to a laboratory for analysis.

Dysfunctional uterine bleeding (DUB): Excessive uterine bleeding.

Endometrial cancer: A malignancy that affects cells lining the uterus.

Endometrial hyperplasia: A condition marked by thickening of the uterine lining (overgrowth of cells in the endometrium) that may cause excessive bleeding.

Endometrial polyps: Small benign growths that protrude into the uterus.

Endometrial ablation: An outpatient procedure that may involve using a laser to eliminate the cells lining the uterus. The procedure may make conception possible.

Endometriosis: A reproductive system disorder in which tissue from the inner lining of the uterus grows in places it should not be. Endometrial tissue can implant itself anywhere in the pelvic area (including the ovaries, bladder, and large intestine), leading to scar tissue and pain during sexual intercourse and bowel movements. Some patients report a constant dull pain in the abdomen, and an escalation in the degree of pain during menstruation.

Endometrium: The inner lining of the uterus.

Epidural: A procedure in which nerves are numbed from the waist down.

Estrogen: A hormone formed by the ovaries, the placenta during pregnancy, and, to a lesser extent, fat cells with the aid of an enzyme called aromatase. Estrogen stimulates secondary sex characteristics, such as the growth of breasts, and exerts systemic effects (i.e., growth and maturation of long bones and control of the menstrual cycle).

Fallopian tubes: Also known as the oviducts. Located at the top part of the uterus (the fundus), the fallopian tubes are the conduits through which eggs cells (ova) are transported to the uterus. At their uppermost ends, the tubes have fingerlike projections that sweep eggs from the ovaries. Each tube measures about four inches in length and possesses contractile capability, a motion that allows them to propel an egg into the uterus.

Follicle cells: A type of cell located in the ovary that produces eggs.

Follicle-stimulating hormone (FSH): Produced by the pituitary gland in the brain; when suppressed by estrogen, FSH inhibits ovulation in the earlier phase of the menstrual cycle.

Gonadotropin-releasing hormone (GnRH) agonists: A group of medications that prevents the body from making estrogen and progesterone. These medications can be prescribed to help to reduce the size of fibroid tumors by creating a state of pseudomenopause.

Gynecologic oncologist: A gynecologist who has completed a post-residency fellowship in diagnosing and treating cancers of the female reproductive organs.

Gynecologist: A medical doctor who has completed a residency specializing in disorders of the female reproductive tract and issues involving endocrinology and reproductive physiology.

Hereditary predisposition: Suggests the likelihood that a medical condition has a familial link.

Hormone replacement therapy (HRT): Medication containing one or more female hormones. HRT is most often used to treat symptoms of menopause, including hot flashes, vaginal dryness, mood swings, sleep disorders, and decreased sexual desire. Estrogen replacement therapy is a form of HRT that includes only the estrogen hormone.

Hysterectomy: The surgical removal of the uterus.

Hysteroscopy: A diagnostic procedure that uses a telescopic instrument to inspect the uterus.

Immune system dysfunction: A theory of endometriosis that suggests the disorder results from the immune system's failure to destroy any endometrial cells remaining after menstruation.

Informed consent form: A legal document that explains any invasive medical procedure, which must be read and signed by the patient in advance. Most forms describe the procedure and indicate that you have been informed of its risks and benefits.

Interligamentous fibroid: A type of growth that develops within a ligament that supports the uterus in the pelvic area.

Interventional radiologist: A medical doctor who has completed a residency in radiology and post-residency training in interventional radiology.

Intramural fibroid: A type of fibroid that grows between the smooth muscular walls of the uterus. It may cause symptoms similar to those of submucosal and subserosal fibroids.

Laparoscope: A very small, thin surgical instrument that allows inspection of the abdominal organs through a tiny camera attached to the device.

Laser: A high-energy light source that emits a beam in a specified wavelength. A laser can quickly vaporize abnormalities with its heat.

Menorrhagia: Heavy menstrual bleeding within a normal cycle; may be a symptom of dysfunctional uterine bleeding.

Menstruation: A discharge of blood, secretions, and tissue fragments from the uterus at regular intervals, usually after ovulation.

Metaplasia: A theory of endometriosis suggesting that endometrial islands are deposited outside of the uterus before birth, during the earlier phases of fetal development. As an adult, these deposits attempt to function as if they, too, are a uterus.

Metrorrhagia: Bleeding between menstrual periods. This may be a symptom of dysfunctional uterine bleeding.

Mifepristone: A synthetic steroid hormone that blocks the action of progesterone. It is used in a few small studies of women with fibroids and is capable of slowing or sometimes stopping fibroid growth.

Myolysis: A surgical procedure in which the blood supply to fibroids is halted, causing them to shrink and die.

Myomectomy: A type of surgery used to remove an individual fibroid.

Nonsteroidal anti-inflammatory drugs (NSAIDs): A group of medications (aspirin, ibuprofen, and naproxen) that reduce inflammation and simultaneously affect the natural hormone-like fatty acids known as prostaglandins, which are a major source of pain and inflammation.

Oophorectomy: Removal of the ovaries. This can trigger the immediate onset of menopause and menopausal symptoms, including hot flashes, night sweats, mood swings, vaginal dryness, and short-term memory loss.

Osteopenia: A condition of decreased calcification or density of bone.

Ovary: Twin oval-shaped glands about the size of an almond. They are located on either side of the uterus and contain thousands of ova, also known as germ cells. One egg is released per month, starting at puberty and continuing in a clocklike pattern throughout most of the reproductive years.

Parasitic fibroid: A growth that develops outside of the uterus, such as on the pelvic wall.

Partial hysterectomy: The surgical removal of the pear-shaped uterus, leaving the cervix in place.

Pedunculated fibroids: A type of fibroid that grows on a stalk usually on the outside of the uterus.

Pelvic congestion syndrome: A disorder in which the veins that nourish the uterus widen, thus causing blood to pool and resulting in debilitating pain.

Pelvic inflammatory disease (PID): Acute or chronic inflammation of female pelvic structures (endometrium, uterine tubes, and pelvic peritoneum) due to infection (gonorrhea, chlamydia, and other organisms). If left untreated, PID can result in scarring and infertility.

Pelvic pressure: A sensation of fullness in the abdomen that can be caused by fibroids.

Pelvic ultrasound: A machine that utilizes ultrasonic waves to take pictures of the uterus, fallopian tubes, and ovaries, and is used as a diagnostic tool by the doctor. The diagnostic pictures may be taken through the abdomen or through the vagina.

Perimenopause: A stage in a woman's life when the ovaries no longer function as in youth; precursor of menopause.

Pessary: A plastic device that, when placed in the vagina, helps to support the uterus.

Polymenorrhea: Menstrual periods that occur far too frequently, usually within a cycle of less than 21 days. This may be a symptom of dysfunctional uterine bleeding.

Progesterone: A sex hormone that prepares the uterus for pregnancy.

Prostaglandins: A family of potent hormone-like fatty acids secreted by an array of tissues that can serve as a source of pain and inflammation. Prostaglandins have been implicated in a wide variety of pain syndromes from migraine headaches to uterine cramps.

Rectovaginal examination: A type of investigation used for diagnosis, in which the physician simultaneously places one lubricated gloved finger in the vagina and another in the rectum. This is an important test for pelvic abnormalities.

Retrograde menstruation: A theory that endometriosis is a process of reverse menstruation in which, instead of flowing out of the body, the blood backs up into the reproductive system, moving into the fallopian tubes and elsewhere throughout the pelvic region. Instead of being discarded as menstrual waste, this residue from the uterus deposits itself throughout the pelvic area and continues to bleed and function as if it were still lining the uterus.

Sarcoma: A highly malignant type of tumor; connective tissue neoplasm.

Serosa: Thin outer layer that covers the uterus.

Simple endometrial hyperplasia with atypia: A term used by pathologists for cells that demonstrate an abnormality and possess about an 80% chance of becoming cancerous. The usual recommendation for patients is a D&C, progestin therapy, and periodic monitoring.

Simple hyperplasia: A condition typified by an overgrowth of cells in the uterus causing the inner lining of the uterus to become thickened. Despite such cellular proliferation, the uterine structure remains unchanged and there is no evidence of atypical or precancerous cells. Also called mild, Swiss cheese, and cystic hyperplasia.

Submucous or submucosal fibroid: A type of fibroid tumor that develops directly beneath the surface of the endometrium. The large number of blood vessels on its surface can bleed and trigger pain. These fibroids tend to prevent the uterine muscle's ability to properly contract because they distort the shape and function of the organ. They can grow to a size that obstructs the fallopian tubes and also may distort the uterine lining as they grow, causing menstrual irregularities. They may even become pedunculated and project into the cervix or vagina.

Subserosal fibroids: Fibroids located beneath the outer covering or outer layer (serosa) of the uterus.

Total abdominal hysterectomy with bilateral salpingo-oophorectomy (TAH-BSO): A type of hysterectomy that involves the removal of the uterus, fallopian tubes, and both ovaries.

Total hysterectomy: The surgical removal of the uterus and cervix.

Transmural fibroids: Fibroids located within the muscular wall of the uterus. Some of the larger fibroids may extend from the innermost layer (submucosa) of the uterus to the outermost layer (serosa). These would be described as transmural fibroids, which have a submucosal and a subserosal component.

Ultrasound: A type of imaging machine that use high frequency sound waves for medical diagnoses.

Urinary incontinence: An inability to prevent the excretion of urine.

Uterine artery embolization (UAE): A surgical technique that blocks the blood supply to problematic fibroids.

Uterine fibroids: Benign tumors that can cause severe abnormal bleeding and extreme pain. Also known as fibromyoma, leiomyoma, and myoma. They may trigger heavy menstrual bleeding, disabling cramps, unpredictable bleeding between periods, and may underlie serious anemia and exhaustion.

Uterine prolapse: Also known as pelvic relaxation, this condition occurs when the ligaments that hold the uterus and/or bladder in place loosen. Severe weakening may allow the organ(s) to protrude through the vagina.

Uterus: Also called the womb. This is a pear-shaped hollow organ about three inches long and two inches wide at its top. It has a role in the monthly menstrual cycle, provides an environment for the growth and nourishment of a developing fetus, and produces mild contractile waves as part of the female sexual response.

Vagina: The passageway from outside of the body to the interior of the reproductive system.

Vaginal hysterectomy: Type of surgery that removes the uterus through the vagina.

Vascular and/or lymphatic transport: A theory of endometriosis in which endometrial implants are carried to inappropriate sites in the body via the bloodstream, the lymphatic system, or both.

Index